DR.
CANTOR'S
LONGEVITY
DIET:

How

to

Slow

Down

Aging

and

Prolong

Youth

and

Vigor

———◆———

Alfred J.
Cantor
M.D.

Parker Publishing Company, Inc.   West Nyack, N.Y.

Author's Previous Books

RIDDING YOURSELF OF PSYCHOSOMATIC HEALTH WRECKERS

UNITROL: THE HEALING MAGIC OF THE MIND

AND TEN OTHERS

Third Printing . . . October, 1968

PRINTED IN THE UNITED STATES OF AMERICA
B&P

For
Eleanor, Alfred Jay, and Pam
With all my love

ACKNOWLEDGMENTS

My special gratitude, as always, goes to Eleanor, Pam and Jay for their constant encouragement and their expert editorial and typing assistance.

It is my special hope that this book will extend the teachings of UNITROL and bring further hope, comfort and longer life to all its students throughout the world.

Prepared under the auspices of UNITROL Teaching Institute, 147-41 Sanford Avenue, Flushing, New York, 11355.

INTRODUCTION

Ponce de Leon, the fifteenth century Spanish explorer, searched for years for the fabled Fountain of Youth, that legendary spring supposed to restore the youth and health of anyone who drank from it. However, de Leon's search was in vain. Although man has always longed for a magically rejuvenating process, he has, nevertheless, grown more sophisticated since the time of de Leon. Today, the suggestion of a search for a Fountain of Youth would arouse only jeers and ridicule from most people.

Nevertheless, the Fountain of Youth does exist! It has been found —not in any remote or unexplored region of the world, but in the laboratories of medical science!

What Medical Science Has Discovered

For the past several years medical science has been studying the ailments and problems of "aging." Its conclusions may be stated as follows: There are no such ailments and problems. There are no diseases that occur just because of the passage of a certain number of years in a person's life. Most illnesses and body deterioration are dependent on certain environmental factors. Therefore, conditions of illness and deterioration can be "modified" by changing and controlling the environment for a person.

Now, from our standpoint, yours and mine, just what is the

major, controllable environmental factor to be modified or changed
in order to gain a healthful long life? You can say it in one word—
NUTRITION.

Dr. Cantor's Key Program—Your Personal Fountain of Youth

For the first time anywhere, this book presents to you my personal health program, featuring the Longevity Diet. It describes
the Cantor Cocktail, vitalizing minerals, and other proven keys to
bountiful good health for a long life. It also includes benefits based
on over 31 years of my own private practice of medicine and the
successful treatment of many hundreds of patients (several of whose
case histories appear in this book), and tells you about my *own*
personal fight for life and renewed health after a serious and lingering illness.

You Can Live Longer, Look Younger, Feel Youthful

The immediate benefits of the *Longevity Diet* seem almost miraculous. Within a very short time this amazing dietary program
can begin to turn back the biological clock for you. The tell-tale
signs of age disappear, your skin clears and takes on a youthful
glow, and you look years younger.

And, at the same time, you feel younger. Gone is the tired,
dragged-out feeling, the lack of pep and energy. Suddenly you feel
capable of anything! You are a happier, more vibrant person—one
able to really enjoy living again.

And you have so much living to do—for your life is just beginning! The *Longevity Diet* can add many, many years to your life.
An age of 100 plus is your birthright, and with the help of the
Longevity Diet you are now able to claim this heritage. But these
added years will not be empty, useless years—a time of lingering
pain and misery; they will be a vigorous time, a time to live life to
the fullest and enjoy every minute of it.

Revitalization: The Secret Benefit

The secret benefit of this book's health program is the revitalization of body tissues and organs. In truth, not only will you look

younger, not only will you feel younger, *you will actually be younger*. Tissues and organs will become more resistant to disease and better able to delay degenerative changes.

Chronic diseases, particularly those that attack the lungs and kidneys, are especially slowed by this dietary program, as is the development of tumors. The *Longevity Diet,* combined with the other Keys to Longevity, serves to control high blood pressure, diabetes, and other serious problems. With this program it may be possible to delay, prevent, and even reverse atherosclerosis, and thus reduce the ravages of today's Number One Killer—heart and blood vessel disease. Your mental powers increase; your personality sparkles. And, as an added benefit, you *naturally* correct any weight problem you may have, automatically and effortlessly—while you eat well!

Simple, Easy-to-follow Directions

There is nothing complex and difficult about the Cantor Program. It offers each individual an easy-to-follow, step-by-step program. It is not set up in stiff medical terminology that requires a doctor's training to understand. It is written for lay people. It is written for you.

Begin Now to Change Your Life by Using This Book

Begin now to change your life. Free yourself from pains, aches, and ailments. Gain new vigor, keep young in body, mind and spirit. Become stronger. Overcome fatigue. Prevent premature old age from creeping up on you. You will have more energy and pep. You will gain a new zest for living. You will feel younger, look younger, and enjoy a happier, healthier, *longer* life.

Alfred J. Cantor, M.D.

What this book
will do for you

This book is different from any other book you have ever read. It provides a "one-two-three-four, step-by-step" method to help you STAY YOUNG FOR A LONGER LIFE, and teaches a simple and successful way for you to use the Cantor Program for Constant Youth. This program consists of Four Keys to Health and Longevity. When you have learned to use these Four Keys, you will have unlocked the long sought secrets of the ages, and you will have found the formula for renewed health and longer life.

What is this magic-like formula? You will find it in the Four Keys of this single volume. *The First Key to Longevity, your first step to staying young for a longer life, is the Nutritional Key.* We know that the major cause of death is heart and artery disease. This First Key to Longevity closes the doors to heart and artery disease at the same time that it opens the doors of longer life and renewed youth. Obviously, if we can cut down on the frequency of heart and artery disease, we can prolong our lives for many years; and—I bring you good news! This *can* be done. The First Key to Longevity shows you how. It is a very simple procedure, requires no drugs, and you will enjoy doing it.

The Second Key to Longevity is the Key to rejuvenation of your general body tissues, as well as your heart and arteries. The secret is found in "fun" forms of pleasantly stimulating exercise. It also unlocks the dynamic secrets of the subconscious, and shows you how to combine the infinite power of your subconscious mind with the only natural exercise *to make you younger, slimmer, and more attractive.*

These two Keys work together just like the two keys of a safety deposit box, one held by you and the other held by the bank. But, wonder of wonders, you hold both Keys in your own hands when you hold this book.

The Third Key to Longevity introduces you to the magically acting hormones. You will learn what hormones are, how they are produced, and what they can do to keep you young for a longer life. You will get to know about the sexual revolution, and you will be detoured around or brought back from the neuter "third" sex. Women will be taught the secret of combined birth and age control. Both men and women will learn the secret of constant youth, and will secure the benefits of hormone heart insurance.

The Fourth Key to Longevity—a truly magical Key—shows you how to rejuvenate your mind. This is the Key that locks the door on early senility of the mind while opening the door to youthful and dynamic patterns of thinking. You are not only as old as your arteries, as old as your tissues, as old as your nervous system, as old as your endocrine glands—but, and *most especially, you are as old as you think you are!*

The Fourth Key to Longevity will literally rejuvenate your mind, and you will feel reborn for a triumphant new life. You will learn how to replace the patterns of aging with the patterns of youth. You will learn how to rid yourself of anxiety. You will learn how to enjoy every moment of every day, 365 days a year.

You now know of the Four Keys to health and longevity. You now hold them in your own hands. Use them to unlock the formula for constant youth! I will take your hand every step of the way, and will show you how. I will be your friend, your guide, your physician. We will now take the first step on the path to renewed youth and vigor. We will now turn the First Key to Longevity—together.

CONTENTS

THE SECOND KEY TO HEALTH AND LONGEVITY— THE "FUN" KEY

THE THIRD KEY TO HEALTH AND LONGEVITY— THE HORMONE KEY

THE FOURTH KEY TO LONGEVITY—THE KEY TO THINKING YOUNG CONSTANTLY

YOUR FIRST KEY
TO LONGEVITY

CHAPTER 1

YOU CAN TURN BACK
THE AGING CLOCK

Good News for a Long and Healthy Life!

Good news! You can live a long and healthy life—perhaps you can even live a 100 or a 150 years. Incredible? Yet it is true, and I will show you exactly how to do it as we move along together through this book.

As you read these pages, picture yourself sitting next to my desk in my consulting room. Let me paint the scene for you. Two walls of this room contain overflowing bookshelves, and the other walls are covered with various medical society certificates. You are sitting in a green leather chair to the left of my desk. I am sitting in a red leather chair behind the desk. Your chart is on my desk, and I have just taken your history—the story of your past and present problems. You are at ease, and we are friends.

As you read through the pages of this book, think of us as friends, sitting together in my consulting room. Let this image, and the warm feeling which comes from your knowledge that I want to help you, flood into your mind and heart every time you pick up this book, and throughout each day when you practice my simple teachings.

Your New and Happy Future

Let me tell you what I want to do for you. Regardless of your age and in spite of the problems you now have, I would like to show you how to live a long and productive and happy life. I would like to show you how to free yourself from disease. I would like to show you that life can be good, joyous, creative. I would like to give you the necessary know-how for living, the Four Keys to Longevity through better health.

We are starting on a great adventure together, perhaps the most important adventure you will ever have. It will be a safari through the jungles of disease and anxiety, and I promise you that you will learn something from every minute of the journey, for it is the Journey of Life itself that I am talking about.

Your new life, as we adventure together, can be exciting. It can be exhilarating. It can be a golden adventure through time. Up to this point you may have been making the journey from birth to death without ever seeing the scenery. You may have been traveling without zest or spirit, without fun or pleasure. You may have been traveling with the fear of death in your mind and heart every step of the torturous way.

You Will Add Zest to Living

That experience is all over. From this point on you will begin to see the exciting scenery. You will begin to *live* every moment of every hour of every day—365 days a year, and 366 on leap years! From this point on you will learn how to release yourself from fear, and most especially from the ever-present fear of death. You will learn, before we have concluded our adventure together, that you are, in a sense, immortal. And you will learn that the first step toward that immortality is to stay alive as long as possible in your present body. Better still, I will teach you how to do just that.

No Experiments—Only Well-Tested Methods

The ideas I am going to share with you have saved my own life. The method you are about to learn will make your life worth living, just as it has done for me. It is a program that I have developed over the course of more than 30 years of very active medical practice. It has helped thousands of people just like you, and many much worse off than you are, to escape from psychosomatic health wreckers, from daily anxiety, from the dull grind of daily routine and stress. It has helped them to longer and happier living. I hope to do the same for you.

Your Help Is Needed in This Joint Venture

Naturally, I can show you the way, and I intend to go with you—throughout life if you wish. But you must lend a helping hand also as we go along the way to health. There is an old saying that the helping hand you are looking for is at the end of your own arm, and that is so very true! I will show you exactly what to do, step-by-step —one, two, three, four in the magic Four Keys to Longevity, but it is you and you alone who can put this program into action. I can do for you what I have done for thousands of others, but only if you want me to do it, want it with all your heart and desire it with all your soul.

You Don't Have to Be Unhappy About Your Health

Don't resign yourself to a life of unhappiness. You don't have to be unhappy. Remember that the only one who can count you out in the contest ring of life is yourself. And the only one who can pick you up when you have been knocked down is yourself. True, I am here now, and I will help you. But the first thing I want you to do, so I will have a pleasant traveling companion on this life-long journey, is to learn to smile. Try it now. See how much better you feel already.

Why, when you smile your whole face lights up! Your eyes sparkle. You feel better all over. The very act of smiling changes your whole outlook on life, and your body's entire physiology. This is a very important lesson—the lesson of attitudes. *Change your attitude—your way of thinking and feeling about life—and you will change your life.*

You Don't Have to be sick

Nearly all disease is psychosomatic. By this I mean that all disease has a psychic (emotional) component and a somatic (bodily) component. *You have to treat both to get well.* You have to get rid of your fears, your anxieties, and your guilt complexes in order to rid yourself of your emotional disease component. And at the same time, you need the help of your doctor to rid you of the physical body factor, the organic changes.

As a matter of fact, at least 90 per cent (and probably more) of the patients in the average doctor's waiting room have purely emotional problems. Oh, it is true that they will complain of the symptoms of asthma or hay fever, colitis, pain in the chest (the heart!), bone and joint troubles, and a million other things, but the roots of their problems are in their emotions, their fears, their anxieties, and their worries over everyday living. Get rid of those and their "diseases" disappear.

I have described this in great detail in my book, *Ridding Yourself of Psychosomatic Health Wreckers* (Parker Publishing Company, Inc.), and have told my readers exactly how to make themselves well. Read it if you wish, and get rid of your own emotionally based health wreckers. This may be exactly what you need to do as your first step toward a longer and healthier life.

I will tell you a little more about this later, but for the moment we will concentrate on the *First Key to Longevity, the Nutritional Key.*

Premature Aging Can be Stopped

It is really possible for man to live much longer than he does—perhaps for as long as 100 or even 150 years. It is possible to revitalize and rejuvenate those who are aging prematurely. At any age—*at your age*—*you* can be revitalized and your biological or aging time clock can be turned back. Would you be satisfied if we could turn it back ten or 20 years? Would you be happy if we could help you relearn the patterns of your youth? Would you consider your time well spent if we could show you how to make your arteries more flexible, how to get rid of the cholesterol deposits in their linings? Would you like to learn how to revitalize your muscles and joints, how to get around with the bounce and zest of youth? I think you would, and we will try to do just exactly that and more for you right now.

New Youth—at Any Age

I believe that, with the proper effort and direction, you can be revitalized at any age. I believe that the clock can be turned back and rewound so that it will run well for many more years. And I have the experience to prove it. More than that, I have over 1,200 references from medical literature, dealing with both human and animal experiments, to prove it. And very soon, I hope, you will prove it for yourself.

The First Key to Longevity is Proper Diet

All you need to do to start your revitalization processes on their way is to change your eating habits for the better. Simple? You bet it is. The diet that has come to be known as the Cantor Longevity Diet gives you all the simple rules.

But for the moment, all you need to do is to make the change called for in this chapter, and you will be well on your way to renewed youth and better health, as well as longer life.

Coming—A Life Span of 150 Years!

That is the exciting title of an article by Lester David. He makes the following claims, based on studies in this country and abroad:

1. There is no medical or scientific reason why the average man and woman cannot live—comfortably, usefully, and alertly—to the age of 150 or even longer.

2. Impressive evidence is accumulating that the aging process, far from being inevitable, might actually be slowed down and even reversed, so that the body might last twice as long as ordinarily.

That's what he says, and, you know, I heartily agree. I will show you, as we talk to each other in every page of this book, that these claims are not far-fetched, and in fact are well within the realm of possibility for you if you will only follow the easy and effective steps I am about to teach you.

I will not only show you how you can revitalize yourself and extend your life, but I will explain *why* these methods work. I will show you *how* science has proven the truth of these concepts and teachings.

You Can Do What Others Have Done

In my practice I have not only tried to extend the life of the patient, but also the pleasure of living. I wrote a little book that I called, *Immortality—Pathways to Peace of Mind,* to show my patients that there are many roads to immortality, and that they were already traveling one or more of them at that very moment. I showed them how to enjoy life NOW. I released them from the fear of death. I showed them, in that book and in *UNITROL: The Healing Magic of The Mind* (Parker Publishing Company, Inc.), how to rid themselves of their past and present anxieties, their fears, their guilt. I would suggest that you read these books and do the same for yourself. It is quite simple.

I have also been concerned with prolonging or restoring vitality to aging tissues and organs, and note this well: your organs and tissues begin to age from the moment you are born.

My own work and the work of others—both in laboratories and in clinical practice—have convinced me that the potential age limit of man has rarely been approached. Unfortunately, man destroys himself through improper eating, thinking, and living, often damaging his own mind-body unit beyond repair long before he reaches his potential maximum age. And now the time has come to show you some of the scientific laboratory proof that the First Key to Longevity is always *proper eating.*

Scientific Proof of Increased Life-span Through Diet

Imagine yourself in the laboratory of the world-famed nutritionist, Dr. Clive McCay at Cornell University. Dr. McCay studied the effect of growth retardation in fish which were kept on a low protein diet. While conducting this experiment, Dr. McCay observed that trout which were retarded in growth outlived those that grew normally. And so he began experiments on white rats to determine the effect of retarded growth on total life span. Three experiments were conducted, and in all three the diets included an adequate daily allowance of protein, vitamins, minerals, and all other essentials. Retardation of growth was due only to an "inadequate" allowance of calories. Remember this, because it is the golden key to long life. It is the key to revitalization of tissues and internal rejuvenation. *Calories do count! They count against you!*

And now let us return to Dr. McCay and watch his revolutionary experiments. In the first experiment, one group of rats was allowed to grow at a normal rate. Two other groups were retarded in growth by reducing the calorie content of their diet to a bare maintenance level—just enough to maintain life, but not enough to allow growth. Of these two groups, one lived for over 700 days, and the other lived for over 900 days.

What does this mean to you? The normal life-span for this species is about 600 days! The test groups on the limited calories diet lived 700 to 900 days! Let's translate this into human terms. The experimental animals on the low calorie diet added 16.6 per cent to their normal life span at the very least, and 49.8 per cent longer life at their very best. If we assume a rough average of 65 years for the life-span of the average person, and if we were to translate these figures to man, he could expect to live 12 to 36 years longer than he now does *simply by eating less.* That means 77 years at the very least and 101 years at the very best by this one simple change in his eating habits! Good enough? I think so, as a starter.

TAKE NOTICE! ! ! You Can Extend Your Life Span by the Right Diet

From these experiments we can at least conclude that the life-span is flexible, that it can be extended, and that the main factor is diet, especially with regard to eating high-calorie foods. That is certainly obvious, and I hope it makes you sit up and take notice— right now! *Take notice* that you are not predestined to live just so many years and no more. *Take notice* that the number of years you live is entirely up to you. *Take notice* that your life-span can be extended. *Take notice* that the only thing you have to change if you want to live longer is your diet. *Take notice* that, basically, all you have to do is to eat less. How much less? We will get to that a little later, but since I want you to start right now on your First Key to Longevity, the golden Key of Nutrition, the simple rule for you to follow is to eat as little as possible. Begin, then, by eliminating all possible sugars and starches from your diet. These are largely empty calories, dangerous calories, life-shortening calories, *deadly* calories. You don't need them, and you don't want them. You want to live.

And now let's look in again on the eminent Dr. McCay. To avoid possible arguments and criticism, Dr. McCay repeated these experiments many times. For that matter, so did many other researchers in other laboratories. The answer was always the same: retarded growth resulted from a low-calorie diet, resulting in *lengthened youth and lengthened life*. Marvelous? I think it's worth the Nobel Prize.

"Well," you may think, "that's okay for children, but I'm not a child. Besides, retarded growth doesn't sound very good."

The answer is that I would rather be 150 years old and short than six feet tall and dead at an early age. Besides, clinical experience shows that you can overcome this objection by a well-balanced high-protein diet and the right kind of vitamins and minerals, while keeping the total diet at the low caloric level. So much for that problem.

But the experiments start with young animals and you and I are no longer young "animals." True, but the fact is that this will work at any age, especially when combined with the Cantor Cocktail, and the other longevity factors I am going to tell you about as we go along. Let's take it one step at a time. The journey of 1,000 miles begins with but a single step, the Chinese so wisely say. And our journey through time—a journey of 150 years—can only be taken one heartbeat at a time, one moment at a time, one idea at a time. Your first is a simple one, one that you can easily follow right now. *Eat less*. That is your first commandment.

LIMIT CALORIES AND YOU LIMIT DISEASE

I put that all in capital letters because it is so important. This was proven by another researcher, C. M. Jackson. He found that there were fewer lung disorders and middle ear infections in animals whose growth was retarded. It seems that the low caloric diet and the retardation of maturation resulting from it either changes the composition of body tissues and organs so that they are more resistant to infection, or perhaps better equips body tissues to delay the degenerative changes and infections that prematurely end life.

There is very good evidence that the extension of life span in these animals on the magic low caloric diet is due to the slower development of those chronic diseases that produce lung, kidney and middle ear disorders. In fact, one researcher even presented evidence to show that low-caloric diets could restrict the development of tumors.

Diet, Disease and Death

So, you can now see that there is strong scientific evidence—clinical and laboratory evidence—of a direct relationship between the level of caloric intake (the amount and kind of food you eat) and the diseases you suffer from, and how soon you will die.

There is a simple message in all of this—a message for you. You must eat less, reduce your calories, to extend your life and to prevent disease. It is a simple equation: too much food = disease and untimely death. Minimal food = less disease and longer life.

What These Experiments Mean To You!

I have already made it abundantly clear what these experiments mean to you. But this is so important, the meaning is so essential to longer life and less disease, that I want to be absolutely certain that you understand exactly what you must do.

Even if this low caloric diet is started in the middle years, it can and will add both years and vitality to your life. I will show you an excellent example of this a little later in our consultation room discussions. I will tell you the story of the fabulous Luigi Cornaro. For that matter, I will tell you my own story, since I owe my life to the very facts I am recounting here. It worked for me and it will work for you.

You may wonder how experiments with rats have any bearing on human nutrition. The use of these animals in scientific research is quite common, since they are very similar to man in their body functions. So we can apply all the studies described, and the conclusions drawn from them, to you and me. What are these conclusions?

1. Limitation of your calorie intake (the amount and type of food you eat) is all-important if you really want a longer life and greater vitality.
2. Limitation of the amount and kind of food you eat can make your

tissues and organs more resistant to disease and better able to delay degenerative changes.

3. Chronic diseases that attack lungs, kidneys, and the middle ear (the most common location of serious ear infection) are slowed down by a prolonged low calorie diet.

4. The development of some types of tumors is retarded by a low calorie diet.

Is This Diet New?

This advice has been given to us repeatedly throughout the ages. But now we have carefully controlled laboratory experiments to confirm its soundness. And now we have the right kinds of foods to provide a well-balanced, healthful diet even while keeping the calorie content low.

The Luigi Cornaro story is taken from the remote past. But it adds another dimension since it shows how you can start on this routine even in your middle years, and still add both years and renewed creativity and vitality to your life. Cornaro did, and so can you. It seems that Francis Bacon said it well when he wrote, "It seems to be approved by experience, that a spare diet . . . such as is either prescribed by the strict rules of a monastical life, or practiced by hermits, which had necessity and poverty for their rule, *rendereth a man long-lived.*"

Rats—You—and Later Life

And now for the experimental evidence to prove that you can start the Longevity Diet right now, at your present age, and benefit from it. Several doctors studied this question by testing white rats over a period of eight years. These experiments proved that *the degree of body fatness in later life is more important than protein or exercises—especially with regard to length of life.* Rats that became very fat had shorter life-spans than those who were only as much as ten per cent lighter. Now there is something for you to think about! Are you overweight right now? Turn to the table of Optimal Weights (page 144) and find the answer. You may be surprised, even if you have considered yourself to be normal. If you are overweight according to that table, you must reduce the excess if you really want to live longer.

The experiments proved, beyond any doubt, that long life was usual in those rats who were maintained *during the latter half of their life* on a low fat, low starch and sugar diet, in addition to exercise. That statement probably is very important to you, at your present age. It is especially important if you are overweight to any degree, even moderately overweight. And that statement touches on three of the Keys to Longevity—nutrition, obesity control, and exercise.

Best of all, this experiment gives you laboratory proof, the proof of animal experimentation, that no matter what your age, you can prolong your life if you accept and use the First Key to Longevity, the golden Key of Nutrition.

And NOW, in summary . . .

1. You can live 100 years or more.
2. Birthdays don't count, and you can turn back the aging clock.
3. The right foods in the right amounts will help you prevent many chronic diseases, clear those that now exist, and revitalize your tissues and organs.
4. The right foods in the right amounts will help you make your body more disease-resistant and more degeneration-resistant.
5. You are as old as your arteries, and you can rid yourself of the hard deposits in your arteries by following the Longevity Diet.
6. You can delay, prevent, or reverse atherosclerosis (hardening of your arteries) and guard yourself against the number one killer—heart and blood vessel disease.

All you have to do to accomplish all this is to limit the calories in your diet. Begin right now by eliminating sugars and starches as your first step toward longer life and better health.

CHAPTER 2

HOW YOU CAN LIVE
TO BE ONE HUNDRED
AND OVER AND ENJOY
EVERY MINUTE OF IT

*"You will live to be one hundred, and you will enjoy
every minute you are alive."*

That statement came from Dr. Edward L. Bortz, former president
of the American Medical Association, and an expert on the problem
of aging, which is the field of geriatrics. This specialist on diseases of
the aging concluded that our scientists had reached a great breakthrough which would mean "another spectacular extension of the
human life-span" in the next ten or 20 years. He said that in 1962.
Several years have passed since then, and I believe that the breakthrough has already occurred and needs only to be applied.

Practical Bases for Your Reaching One Hundred Years

In this chapter we meet again in my consulting room, and I will
tell you more about the great breakthrough and how you can take
advantage of this opportunity to extend your life. I will also show
you how to enjoy every minute you are alive—not only during this
consultation, but throughout our entire series of visits together.

I will show you that *your arteries are the major key to longer life,* and I will tell you exactly what to do to make them younger again. It is really a very simple dietary rule that I will tell you about. You will enjoy following it, because it is easy and pleasant to manage.

Then I will introduce you to the "magic" minerals. Again, you do not need to take any medicines. Diet alone can turn the trick, and start you on the road to longer life and better health. I will have a great deal more to say about the "magic" minerals later in this book, as we talk together again and again.

I will introduce you to the *mystery mineral.* This is another vital element, a *trace element* that should be included in your diet. It will help in the growth and repair of old and new tissues as you revitalize and restore your body to its new youth.

The Arterial Key to Health and Longer Life

Dr. Bortz was speaking of heart and blood vessel deterioration, and also of cancer, arthritis, and nervous disorders. Heart and artery disease are the major causes of death today. What I am teaching you is how to help prevent heart and artery disease. When you have learned to do this, and when you have controlled the dangerous deposits in your arteries, you will have taken a giant step forward toward a healthier and a longer-lived future.

The final breakthrough has not yet been made for cancer, but advances in the study of nutrition do provide major answers for heart and blood vessel deterioration, our number one killer. There is even the possibility that a proper diet may be important in the prevention or avoidance of certain types of tumors, and perhaps even for the preventive control of cancer.

There is certainly no argument with Dr. Bortz's concluding statement, "We can throw away our canes, crutches, and rocking chairs, if we merely take advantage of what our doctors already know and try to tell us about how to live a century and more." Listen carefully as I tell you how to do just that as we meet in our consulting room visits.

You Are as Old as Your Arteries

Since man is as old as his arteries, and since heart and arterial disease are the number one killers, your attack must be directed

against diseases of the arteries to attain longer life. I will give you
all the ammunition you need for this attack in the modern concepts
of nutrition. Take heart! (and that is more than a pun)—*simple dietary changes will prevent hardening of your arteries* caused by the
deposit of cholesterol in their walls. In fact, you may even reverse the process and *get rid* of the cholesterol deposits that now
clog your arteries and threaten your very life! Atherosclerosis is the
killer disease in which fatty deposits on the walls of the arteries reduce the flow of blood. This makes it more likely that we will develop blood clots, perhaps even the frightening and often fatal
coronary thrombosis.

The Second Secret of Prevention of Heart and Blood Vessel Diseases for Longer Life

I will now tell you the simple second secret for the prevention of
heart and blood vessel disease. You will remember that the first secret, the rule relating to the First Key to Longevity, was to reduce
your total caloric intake (eat less starch and sugars). The second
secret is to reduce the amount of *saturated fats* in your diet. I will
have much more to tell you about this in a later consultation, but I
want to introduce you to this important golden Key of Nutrition so
you can begin immediately to restore your own arteries to normal,
to youth.

We now know that there is a close relationship between the highly
saturated fats, the fats found in meat, butter and dairy products, and
atherosclerosis. These are the animal fats, and it almost seems as
though man is being killed in return when he kills and eats animals.
This is part of the balance of nature, of course, but it need not be so.
All you have to do to prevent these saturated fat deposits in your
arteries is to avoid these animal fats as if they were poison.

I am not necessarily recommending a vegetarian diet for you, and
I am not myself a vegetarian. But if you did eliminate the animal fats
completely, you would be doing yourself a good turn. Still, since
most of us enjoy eating meat and drinking milk, and since most of us
like both eggs and butter, I want you to know a few simple rules to
help you over this diet hurdle without doing any harm to your arteries and your heart.

The Caution Signals In Eating Fats of Various Types

Your first rule is to limit the amounts of animal fats that you eat. And here is an interesting fact: the "best" steaks, sold in the high-priced, fancy steak houses, are the most dangerous from the fat content point of view. They are heavily "marbled," which means that there is much fat in the layers between the red meat. If you order your steak rare (and most of us who are steak-eaters like our meat rare) *the fat is not cooked out.* This makes these "best" steaks literally the worst for your heart and arteries! They are full of the killer—*saturated fat.* The lesson to be learned from this is simply to buy cheaper cuts of steak, and cook them well to drain off the fat. It is best to learn to like your steak well-done, if you must eat steak.

The next rule is to eat small portions. Don't order the big cuts of steak and beef, the "Diamond Jim Brady" portions. Remember that his appetite killed him at a very early age!

As to milk, learn to like skimmed milk. I have learned to enjoy skimmed milk, although I only use it in my Cantor Cocktail (more about that later). Stay away from the fat-rich regular milk and cream. There are vegetable substitutes for milk that can be used in your coffee, and taste quite good. They are free from saturated fats.

What about eggs? One or two a week probably will not kill you. There are even eggs now available from chickens who have been given a special feed so that the fat and cholesterol content of their eggs is much reduced. I myself like the whites of eggs, and I eat two each morning, throwing away the hard boiled yolks.

Why You Should Replace Saturated Fats with Unsaturated Fats

There are relatively simple ways to replace the saturated fats by equivalent products that are highly unsaturated (polyunsaturated fats). The polyunsaturated fats are protective to your arteries, and when you reduce the saturated fats in your food and substitute the highly unsaturated fats, you hasten the departure of the cholesterol deposits in your arteries. At the same time, the level of cholesterol in your blood will most probably return to normal. In this way, you not only prevent further deposits of cholesterol in your already congested or narrowed arteries, but also rid yourself of the present blockage in your blood vessels.

Now let's see just exactly how you are to do this. Let us take butter as an example. There are polyunsaturated margarines now available in every grocery store and supermarket, margarines made from corn oil or safflower seed oil. Read the label, and if it tells you that the margarine is produced from polyunsaturated corn or safflower seed oil, and is only partially hydrogenated, you may use this product on your bread or for frying. You may use it safely for better health.

Warning About Hydrogenated (Hardened) Margarine

If the margarine is very solid, however, it may be very hydrogenated and very dangerous. When hydrogen is added to corn or safflower seed oil, the oil becomes more solid, but at the same time it becomes more saturated *(for that is what saturated means—saturated with hydrogen, just like natural butter)*. Obviously, liquid oils are quite unsaturated, and fats that are solid at room temperature are usually quite saturated and dangerous to your heart and arteries. The Cantor Cocktail, which I will tell you about later, takes skimmed milk and reconstitutes it to its previous form by adding the highly unsaturated safflower oil to replace the natural fat that had been removed at the dairy. See page 164 for details.

How Cholesterol Chokes Your Arteries

For a simple example, think of automobile engine lubrication. If the amount of carbon and impurities is low, the oil flows smoothly and the engine performs efficiently. However, as excess carbon and "sludge"—gummy deposits—get into the oil, these are deposited on vital parts of the engine, causing wear and destruction. The same thing happens in your blood circulation system. If the cholesterol level is low—as it should be—there are no deposits of this fatty wax on, and in, your artery walls, and the blood flows smoothly and freely to all your tissue structures. Since your blood carries all the vital tissue nutrients, this smooth flow is essential for normal tissue growth and repair. It is also essential for normal tissue function to keep you alive and healthy.

But if your blood cholesterol level rises abnormally, cholesterol is then deposited out of the circulating blood on and in your artery walls, blocking the normal flow of blood. Your blocked arteries become narrowed, and the obstructed thin stream of blood might easily clot in these blocked vessels. If this happens in the heart arteries, we call it a coronary thrombosis—a serious form of heart attack. If this blockage occurs in a brain blood vessel, the result is a "stroke."

How to Prevent or Avoid This Blocking in Your Blood Vessels

Fortunately—as you already know—this blocking can be prevented or effectively coped with. These deposits can be cleaned out of your partially blocked blood vessels and further deposits can be avoided.

Since most adult American males have some degree of atherosclerosis, and since these deposits actually begin in early childhood(!)—it is very important to know how to avoid and clear up this deadly problem of blocked arteries. After the menopause, most American women begin to develop the same condition.

It is obviously of enormous importance for all of us to learn how to avoid, prevent, and reverse artery blockage of normal blood circulation. The way to reduce cholesterol in your blood and in your arteries is to learn the new concepts of nutrition, step-by-step, as you and I discuss them in our consulting room sessions. The nutritional principles you are learning will get rid of the "rust" in your artery "plumbing system." But these principles will do this for you only if you put them into action immediately. I would suggest that you *do this one step at a time*. For example, your first consultation taught you the enormous importance of reducing the amount of food you eat. I suggested that you promptly eliminate sugars and starches from your diet. Have you done this? If you have not, *begin right now*. Each day that goes by allows your body and your arteries to grow older and older, bringing you closer and closer to the danger point of heart or artery disaster. So START NOW. REDUCE CALORIES IN YOUR DIET.

Do this for one week. Certainly that is not asking too much. Do it one day at a time. You can do it for one day, can't you? When that day is over, you need only do it for one day more, when the next day comes. And so on, for one week at a time. Soon you will find it easier and easier, and then you will enjoy the obvious revitalization, the new energy, the new face and figure, the new YOU.

The second week of your Longevity Program I would like you to eliminate the solid animal fats, the dairy fats, and to substitute the polyunsaturated oil—exactly as instructed above. That is very simple, and certainly no sacrifice. All right, let us assume that your second week is here. One day at a time, the easy way, add the low fat (all polyunsaturated) rule to the low calorie rule of the previous week.

Another Note of Caution on Fats

Remember that fat is very high in calories. The less you take the better, if you are to stay with your low calorie rule. So I now give you the outside limit for the polyunsaturated fats, the ones that help you eliminate cholesterol and safeguard your arteries and heart.

You are to drink three ounces of safflower oil each day. You may put this oil on salads, with lemon juice or vinegar, and you may add garlic to taste if you want a wonderful French dressing. Or you may take your oil straight, drinking it without embellishment. Or—and this is the way I take it—you mix the Cantor Cocktail and drink it before each meal. This has many advantages. One advantage is the fact that this mixture reduces your appetite if taken just before meals. *That makes it easier to eat less*—remember your low calorie rule.

The "Magic" of the Safflower Oil Cocktail (Cantor Cocktail)

Fats make you feel full. This is called the "satiety" value of a food, and this appetite-satisfying value is highest for fats, much higher than for proteins or starches or sugars.

Fats slow the emptying time of the stomach. The longer food remains in your stomach, the longer it will be before you feel hungry again. For that matter, I doubt that most of us know what real hunger feels like. We eat as a result of habit—the clock is our guide and not hunger. This is unnatural eating, an unnatural pattern, and anything that is unnatural is potentially dangerous.

The final "magic" of the Cantor Cocktail is, of course, the magic that it works in your heart and arteries. Believe me, if nutritional studies had nothing more remarkable than cholesterol control and the low calorie concept to offer, it would still represent a truly major contribution to health and life extension in this century!

Your Life May Be Saved by This Simple Dietary Change!

There is no doubt that millions of lives can be saved by such simple dietary changes. And there is still more good news to come, as we talk together!

There is no doubt that the human life span can be extended to a minimum of a 100 years by the same simple diet changes combined with the other advice I have yet to give you.

And there is still more to tell you in this same consultation, for we have yet to talk about the "magic" minerals, another contribution of nutrition to longer life and healthier arteries.

All I ask you to remember is that the life you save may well be your own. Make it your own to start with, and then pass on these teachings to your family and friends. After all, there is less point in staying alive 100 or more years if you are to be alone. Keep your family and friends with you throughout this long life and enjoy it together.

The "Magic" Minerals

I want to take you now to the University of Rochester's School of Medicine and introduce you to William H. Strain, Ph.D., another distinguished researcher. Dr. Strain's work shows that minerals from the ancient Permian Seas (about 200,000,000 years ago) may determine how long you will live.

His carefully developed statistics and clinical findings show that there is a widespread deficiency of two minor elements, vanadium and zinc, in the average man's diet. Now here is the reason why this is important to you—*vanadium checks, and can prevent cholesterol development in the human body.*

Now you want to know where you can get vanadium, and I am anxious to tell you. Vanadium is found in the drinking water of certain areas of the Southwest. In these areas the death rates from cardiovascular problems are very low, much lower than in the rest of our country. These regions were once covered by the Permian Seas, and as a result the drinking water is "hard" or mineralized. Incidentally, I think this is one of the major reasons why that natural Shangri La, Hunza-Land of the Himalayas—where men and women commonly live active lives well beyond a hundred, is a haven of outstanding longevity and vigor. There, waters are fed by ancient glaciers and are heavily mineralized from deposits accumulated over millions of years. Vanadium is not found in appreciable amounts in the "soft" waters of the Coastal and Great Lakes States of our country, and in these areas the death rates from cardiovascular problems are higher than in the Southwest. The relationship certainly seems obvious.

How Does Vanadium Work?

It seems that vanadium, taken in proper amounts, results in a reduced accumulation of cholesterol in our artery walls. In fact, Dr. Strain says that there are other benefits as well. "Proper dietary intake of vanadium," he claims, "may give lower cholesterol content of the skin, *reduce the incidence of gall stones, and lessen accumulation of cholesterol in the arterial walls.*"

The work of other scientists has also shown that the "harder" the water (the higher the mineral content), the lower the number of deaths from heart and blood vessel disease, especially those deaths due to high blood pressure and atherosclerosis (hardened arteries from cholesterol deposits).

Dr. Strain's work is well substantiated and documented, if not proven beyond a doubt. This is truly remarkable! You now know that the next step in your Longevity Diet is to obtain the proper amounts of dietary minerals, especially the wonderful qualities of vanadium.

Hard Water Is Good For Your Health

It is now obvious to you that "hard" water is truly good for you, no matter how it tastes. If you are lucky enough to live in the naturally mineralized areas of the Southwest, you have no problem. In other areas, you will have to supplement your underprivileged water to stay alive as long as possible. Since hard water contains minerals that are not only necessary but also vital, to reduce your chances of becoming a cardiac statistic, we must find out where to get the vital vanadium.

How to Upgrade or Supplement "Underprivileged" Water Through Simple Diet Changes

Now here is the answer you have been waiting for. No drugs! The answer is found in natural foods. For those of you who live in the "underprivileged" water areas, as I do, you will be happy to know that both vanadium and zinc are found in certain ocean fish, especially *sardines and herring*. All you have to do is add these ocean fish to your daily diet to reduce cholesterol accumulation in your arteries, to help stop the formation of gall stones, and even to improve your skin texture. Your first specific item in the Longevity Diet (after the safflower oil) is ocean fish and plenty of it—especially sardines and herring. But please don't take them heavily salted or smoked. Try to get them in their natural state. Too much salt is dangerous, especially for heart and high blood pressure problems, and smoked food may somehow be related to cancer. Fair warning!

The Mystery Mineral—Zinc

Zinc is a mystery mineral, perhaps even more mysterious than vanadium. We do not yet know very much about the importance and function of zinc in the human body. It seems to be essential for growth and repair of tissues. It may also be necessary for proper gall bladder function, and even for normal arterial structure.

In any case, it is what we call a vital mineral trace element and should be included in your Longevity Diet for obvious reasons. I will tell you about more magic minerals in our next consultation. I will also tell you more about the mystery of the sardine. But now I want to keep a promise I made at the beginning of this consultation when I promised to tell you not only how to live longer, but also how to enjoy every moment of your life.

Here are Your Tips for Better Living . . .

1. Learn to forgive yourself for your past "sins" and "mistakes." When you do this you will be born anew each day of your life. Won't

it be wonderful to start each day fresh, a new person in a fresh, new world?

2. Learn to respect and love yourself. Only then can you love others.

3. Learn how to be selfish and look after yourself. Only then can you be generous and look after others.

4. Learn how to seek out new experiences, new friends, and new ideas each day of your life. Be as creative as you can, for this is the hallmark of youth, and youth is what you want to regain or keep.

5. Smile, if you want to feel good. Do it right now, and see how much better it makes you feel. Get the *smile habit*.

6. When the going gets rough, keep smiling and keep punching. Never give up. You are the only one who can count you out.

7. Try to turn defeat into victory by staying with your problems until they are resolved. Dale Carnegie said it well when he told us, "When Fate hands you a lemon, make lemonade." Easier said than done? Sure, but you can do it better each day as you become truly younger and younger in body and mind.

8. Learn to be content with what you have (while working like the very devil to improve your circumstances!).

The Talmud tells us that *the man who is content with what he has is truly rich*.

9. Learn to accept whatever cannot be changed, and learn to live with it.

10. Above all, remember that life is made up of very fleeting present moments. If you don't live life RIGHT NOW, soon there will be no more present moments to live.

So start right now to have fun. Today is your day. Tomorrow is still another today, and I want you to fill each today, each tomorrow as it becomes a today—with FUN.

When the late and great President, John F. Kennedy, was asked what he regretted most, he said that he regretted not having had more good times. We are a long time dead. HAVE FUN NOW.

There you have some of the answers to how to enjoy life. Put them to work NOW. NOW is the key word, and the rest is up to you.

And NOW, in summary . . .

In this important chapter you have learned—

1. You can live to be a hundred and enjoy every minute you are alive.

2. Your arteries are the major key to longer life and better health.

3. You have learned that you are as old as your arteries, and that your arteries can be made young again.

4. You have learned the secret of prevention of hardening of the arteries by cholesterol deposits.

5. You have learned that you must reduce the total fat content of your diet, especially by eliminating the animal and dairy fats.

6. You have learned the very tasty substitutes, and the secret of the polyunsaturated oils.

7. You have learned about the Cantor Cocktail and how it helps your heart and arteries, reduces your appetite, and keeps you young in many other ways.

8. You have learned how cholesterol does its damage, and how you can prevent and undo that change.

9. You have been given the first important elements of a one-step-at-a-time, one-day-at-a-time, one-week-at-a-time Longevity Program—the easy way to live longer and better.

10. You have learned about the magic minerals, and where to find them. They will help you stay alive and healthier *in a simple and pleasant way*—another secret of the First Key to Longevity.

11. And finally, I have kept my promise by giving you some tips on how to enjoy life. Follow them and you will find that *life can be fun!*

CHAPTER 3

YOUR LEGACY OF
"MAGIC MINERALS"
FROM ANCIENT OCEANS

Once again we find ourselves together in my consulting room. Make yourself comfortable and we will continue our journey together into longer life and greater vitality. Up to this point you have learned a great deal. You now know that you can live to be 100 or more years of age, and that you can keep your body in tip-top condition by making certain relatively simple changes in your eating habits.

These changes will restore your aging arteries to a more youthful condition. The cholesterol deposits that are now narrowing them will begin to depart, leaving your arteries more flexible. Since you are as old as your arteries, this is a giant step forward toward renewed youth and longer life.

The Half-Portion Approach to Eating

You have already started on the first important changes in diet and have reduced your eating calories to a minimum. If you are having trouble with this, remember the simple rule to eliminate, or "skip" starches and sugars that might so craftily tempt you. This will cut a big slice from your usual amount of calories. The next

26

simple logical step is to reduce the size of your portions. Cut them in half. You'll never miss the excess amounts of food you have merely accustomed yourself to eat, and you certainly won't miss the excess pounds of flabby fat you have been carrying about. Each of these free-loading fat pounds contains miles and miles of tiny blood vessels—*the capillaries*—and your heart has to pump blood through each and every inch of them. This is an enormous burden, and simply reducing your weight provides an extra measure of safety and self-help for your heart.

Polyunsaturated versus Saturated Fats

You have also learned that you must substitute polyunsaturated fats for the saturated fats that you may have been eating to excess. You have been told exactly how to do this, and it is very simple indeed. Just eliminate the hard fats of meat and dairy products, and use the very soft (polyunsaturated fats) oils such as safflower oil, safflower oil margarine instead of butter, skimmed milk instead of whole milk, and so forth.

A Drugless, Natural Appetite Depressant

And most important of all—drink the Cantor Cocktail three times a day, one cocktail before each meal. This acts as a natural appetite depressant while providing you with the required amount of the polyunsaturated oil. It does many other things for you, and you can even use these three cocktails as your total food for the day, supplementing them with any vitamin-mineral capsule or tablet your doctor may recommend. If you are not doing heavy manual labor, this will be enough food for you, and you will be fulfilling the Longevity Diet requirements for limiting your calories and also for the polyunsaturated fats.

The "Magic" Minerals' Benefits

You have also learned something about the "magic" minerals, and you now know that you can obtain them in ocean fish, especially the herring family. Simple enough? Just add fish to your diet every day. I hope you like fish. Remember that it is simply a matter of changing your daily habits and you will change your tastes at the same time. As the French say—*habit forms the taste*. Just as with olives, you have to eat quite a few before you get to like them. If you are not yet a fish eater, try fish each day and you will soon get to like the taste, the succulence, the flavor. Best of all, *you are making your arteries younger* and therefore you will become younger.

In this chapter—during this consultation—I intend to tell you still more about the "magic" minerals, and how they will help you renew your youth and prolong your life. I intend to tell you more about Dr. Strain's ideas, and also about the work of my good friend, the famed Montreal researcher, Dr. Hans Selye. You will learn more about the trace elements, especially zinc and vanadium, and a few others, each of them important to your normal health and for the prevention of heart and blood vessel disease.

I will tell you about confirming studies from other parts of the world, the Netherlands, Iceland, England, Africa. And best of all, I will reduce all the experimental work on animals and man to one single simple rule for you to follow—a simple dietary rule, for we are still using the First Key to Longevity, the Nutritional Key.

Your Legacy from Ancient Oceans

And now we are ready to return to Dr. Strain. I want to remind you that he is associated with the University of Rochester School of Medicine and Dentistry. He reached his important conclusions after a study of statistics and clinical findings, and showed that there are widespread deficiencies of *vanadium* and *zinc* in the average American's diet.

He proved that the ancient Permian Seas that once covered certain areas of the South Central and Mountain states contained large amounts of vanadium and zinc. The people of those areas are now the beneficiaries of those ancient seas, for their death rates are, in some respects, very low as compared with other areas.

Your Body and Its Relation to Seawater

If it is true that all life orginated in the ocean, billions of years ago—and there is overwhelming scientific evidence that this is actually so—then it becomes easier for us to understand why fish is so important in our diet. As fish (or some form of ocean life), our most primitive ancestors must have lived on other forms of ocean life. Our bodies are largely water, and 30 per cent of the fluid in our bodies *is essentially dilute seawater!* Remember this important fact when we are building your programs for health. *See how important it is to drink water*—at least six to eight glasses a day, to keep your body tissues from drying out too much? See how important it is to provide your body with the type of minerals found in the ocean?

To maintain this essential internal fluid balance, we must obviously provide ourselves with a diet that contains minerals that duplicate the mineral elements in seawater. If you live in the Permian Sea areas of the United States, or in Hunza-Land of the Himalayas in the Far East, or in certain other world areas where the drinking water is highly mineralized, all you have to do is to drink the water. But if you do not live in these geographical areas, and most of us do not, then you must look elsewhere for these protective trace minerals.

What Are the Important Trace Minerals?

As you know, proteins, fats and carbohydrates are important for human nutrition, but in limited amounts, and of certain kinds (especially the fats). But there are other substances, without energy or food value, that are also vital for growth, for good health and for life itself. These are the mineral salts. The nucleus of tissue cells contains phosphorus. Iron carries, in our blood stream's red corpuscles, the oxygen we cannot live without. Iodine is essential for mental and physical development. A tiny trace of this important mineral makes the difference between a normal mind and that of an imbecile. Most of our minerals are in our bones, especially calcium and phosphorus.

Minerals Cannot Be Stored in the Body

You and I cannot store minerals to any important degree. To avoid deficiencies, *we have to get them every day*. The ones we are most concerned about at this moment are vanadium and zinc (and, as we shall soon see, magnesium and potassium). These are essential for the health of our heart and arteries, and therefore for the prolongation of life.

Benefits of Zinc in Your Diet

You must have enough zinc in your diet and in your body to keep your bones in good shape. If you get enough zinc in your food, your skin will be healthier and all of your body tissues will heal better when they are injured.

Where do you look for zinc? Fish is still the answer, especially sardines and herring. All ocean fish contain vanadium, varying with the species, and some contain both vanadium and zinc. Amazing, isn't it, that simply by eating fish regularly—especially fish of the herring family—you can lower your blood and artery wall cholesterol level, make your arteries younger, help prevent gallstones from forming, and give yourself the fresh and healthy skin of renewed youth and vitality? The amount of fish Scandinavians eat may help explain their longevity, and offers new hope for you and me.

Where Else Can Trace Elements Be Found?

Really, the tremendous importance of the trace elements should come as no surprise to any of us. Iodized salt has been used in this country for over 40 years to combat growth of goiter. The battle over fluoridation of water (adding the trace element, fluoride), for the prevention of dental decay, is known from one end of the country to the other. Iron therapy for "tired blood" was started by the Greeks, long ago. It did not originate with television!

Iodine in the tiniest amount, as I have already told you, may make the difference between an imbecilic and a normal child. Our bodies cannot live and function normally without the trace elements. And they must be literally *trace* in amount, for large amounts can be poisonous.

Very tiny amounts of vanadium are found in vegetables, milk, sea salt, mineralized drinking water, and, of course, in the ocean fish.

Is There Laboratory Proof of the Value of Trace Minerals for the Human Body?

There is laboratory proof that vanadium compounds can reverse experimental hardening of the arteries in rabbits and chickens.

Hardening of the main artery of the body, the aorta, is corrected by feeding vanadium salts to these animals.

A weakened aorta wall is called an aneurysm, and it was an aneurysm that killed the great Albert Einstein. Incidentally, such aneurysms always contain less zinc than normal artery walls, and it may well be that zinc is essential for normal arterial structure. There seems little doubt that we can apply the results of such laboratory studies to man, and draw the necessary conclusions on how to keep ourselves alive and well as long as possible.

What to Do for Trace Element Balance in Your Body

For one thing, as you already know, you can add a variety of ocean fish to your diet for mineral trace balance. Learn to like sardines. Learn to enjoy herrings. Dr. Strain tells us, "The human dietary intake of vanadium is in terms of parts per billion, and animal studies indicate that there is a high factor of safety should vanadium fortification of foodstuffs be instituted." But I see no need for such complicated fortification if you simply add ocean fish to your diet as a health measure.

Sea salt might also be a useful food additive, but you would have to be certain that you do not have high blood pressure or kidney disease. Excessive sea salt (or any other kind of salt) might well be dangerous if you have kidney trouble or a tendency to high blood pressure.

Although the vanadium content of milk varies, milk may also be a good natural source of this important trace mineral.

Just Exactly How Does Vanadium Work?

Laboratory studies show that vanadium prevents cholesterol formation. It does even more, since it hastens the destruction of cholesterol. Even more important is the fact that vanadium lowers the blood cholesterol level. Obviously, the less cholesterol there is in your blood, the less danger there is of deposit of this fatty wax in your arteries. Incidentally, in this country a blood level of up to 250 milligrams of cholesterol is considered normal. But it is also considered normal to die of heart and blood vessel disease in this country. I do not consider the high blood level of cholesterol to be normal, nor do I believe that heart and blood vessel disease should be the number one cause of death in the United States.

More Minerals That Help Your Heart's Health

I promised to tell you something about the remarkable experiments of Hans Selye, experiments that will help you and me to live longer and healthier lives.

Using more than 30,000 experimental rats, and working in his laboratories in the famed University of Montreal, Dr. Selye discovered more magical minerals for the prevention of death of the heart muscle. Under certain experimental conditions, the heart muscle may die as a result of deficiencies in essential minerals such as potassium or magnesium. Potassium and magnesium are essential for good heart muscle health, and they are also important for many other body functions, as well as for the actions of various enzyme systems. Again the magnificent trace minerals in action!

Dr. Selye concluded from his many experiments that treatment or prevention with magnesium and potassium may be the answer for all the various kinds of heart muscle death. Tremendous! Keep our heart muscle healthy and we eliminate much of the number one cause of death!

Should We All Take These Magical Minerals?

We can safely say, as a result of these studies, that heart death from moderate hardening of the arteries by cholesterol deposits seems to be so closely related to the type of experimental heart death Dr. Selye describes, that everyone would benefit from potassium chloride and magnesium chloride. Now let us translate this into simple language for immediate use. All this means that you stand a better chance of staying alive if you get enough magnesium and potassium in your diet.

Magnesium's Mysterious Benefits

In support of this important work by Dr. Selye, a researcher in South Africa, Dr. Bersohn, used magnesium salt for the treatment of coronary patients, with very good results. He found that the

Bantu Negroes, a group relatively free from atherosclerotic heart disease, had higher levels of magnesium in their systems than the white population with advanced atherosclerosis.

Still other researchers have confirmed his findings, and shown that experimental hardening of the arteries could be reduced by taking magnesium. This is enormously important for all of us, and we must make the simple diet changes to include magnesium in our foods.

Not too much is known about potassium in human diet, except that it is another important trace mineral for the prevention of heart and blood vessel disease. For our purposes, that is all we need to know.

Sardines As a Source of Important Minerals For Health

Once again we must return to the lowly sardine for the life-saving, life-prolonging minerals. In just three and one-half ounces of sardines there are about 560 milligrams of potassium, and the recommended requirement of this trace mineral is only 250 milligrams per day. So, for your vanadium, zinc, and potassium you need only look to the sardine. You will get the required amount of magnesium, your other magic mineral, from the basic Longevity Diet, to be fully described during another consultation.

Thoughtful Tips on Enjoying Life More

There is very little point in living 100 or more years unless you learn how to enjoy every minute of every day. Otherwise you will be like the victim of the old gag: "I haven't been married for 50 years yet but it sure seems like it!"

Don't do that to yourself. Learn to enjoy the present moment. Look about you and *see* your family, your friends, your home. Really *see*—become aware of your surroundings in depth. Learn to really *taste* food, and don't simply use your mouth as the gateway to your stomach. Learn to *smell* the falling leaves, the newly mowed grass, the odors of summer, spring, autumn, fall and winter. Learn to smell and enjoy your food as you chew leisurely and happily, one mouthful at a time. Learn to *hear* the sounds around you. Learn to *touch* and *feel*. Learn to *live,* and not simply to *exist.* You are following this book to *live!*

Most of us do not appreciate what we have until it is taken away from us. We don't appreciate the gift of sight until we get a speck of dirt in our eye. We don't appreciate the gift of health until we are ill. We don't appreciate the gift of life until we are ready to die. Learn to count your blessings, and to appreciate each and every one of them right now and each moment of each day.

You come this way but once. Make the most of it. *Stop right now and make a list of your blessings.* Head that list with the first blessing —I AM ALIVE. Now complete the list yourself. Don't go a single step further until you do this. (You'll be glad you did!)

And NOW, in summary . . .

Let's review what we have learned to this point, so you can put your Longevity Program into instant action. You must do this if you are to rid yourself of the aging tissues of your body and replace them with healthier, younger tissues.

1. You have already begun to limit your calories. You are eating half portions, and you have reduced or eliminated sugars and starches from your diet. (It is not possible to eliminate them completely, but you have certainly stopped eating the obvious sugar and starch foods—bread, pies, cakes, pastry, ice cream, candy, spaghetti, and so on.)
2. You have already stopped eating animal and dairy fats, and you are now using the polyunsaturated oils in their place. You are using margarine instead of butter, and you have selected a very unsaturated margarine, preferably one made from safflower oil.
3. You only eat the whites of hard boiled eggs, to avoid the fat and cholesterol in the yolks.
4. You drink your Cantor Cocktail before each meal. This gives you three ounces of safflower oil each day—your full requirement to rid your arteries of their cholesterol deposits.
5. You will now include ocean fish in your *daily diet*. Try to include sardines or herring whenever possible. Use the regular, cheaper grade of sardine, not the skinless and boneless, for sardines are better for you when you get the

minerals of the skin and bones with the rest of the fish. If the sardines come packed in olive oil, drain off the oil after you open the tin, and replace with safflower oil. The taste is indistinguishable, and the health-giving factor is greater (more polyunsaturated).

6. Drink at least six to eight glasses of water each day—preferably hard water (the mineral-containing kind), for hard water has the important trace minerals in it.

7. If you can't get hard water, or have problems with the daily ocean fish requirement, ask your doctor to prescribe a good vitamin-mineral product, one with all the known trace minerals in full dosage.

8. You now know the enormous, life-prolonging properties of the trace minerals, especially vanadium, zinc, magnesium and potassium, and how to get all that your body needs.

9. And finally, I have given you more tips on enjoying life. Since you are preparing to live 100 or more years, you should learn to enjoy every one of them. This is the winning combination. More power to you!

CHAPTER 4

HOW TO AVOID THE NUMBER ONE KILLER— HEART DISEASE

Say "Hello" and "Goodbye" to the Number One Killer

Coronary heart disease is the number one killer, especially of the middle-aged. It is the grim reaper's number one helper for many in the prime of life, especially the business executive, the professional man, and all those under stress. It is also the number one killer of the elderly.

Another frightening fact is that the majority of American males over 25 years of age have atherosclerosis of their coronary arteries —their blood carrying life-lines are reduced in size due to those waxy-fat cholesterol deposits.

Arteriosclerosis (hardening of the arteries) and degenerative disease of the heart account for approximately one-third of all deaths among males in the 45 to 54 age group. Even more astounding, and more disturbing, is the fact that there are—every year—1,000 cases of coronary heart disease for every 100,000 males aged 45 to 54. This is really an epidemic rate, with men dropping like flies!

The tragedy in these figures is even more obvious to you now, since you know that many—if not most—of these deaths could be prevented by proper diet and the other simple rules you will learn as we continue in our consultations together.

Now that you have said hello to the number one killer, you may say goodbye.

How to Say Goodbye to the Number One Killer

You began to say goodbye the minute you picked up this book, the minute you sat down "in my consulting room." You started to say goodbye when you began to follow the rules of the First Key to Longevity. The minute you ate your first half-portion meal, death turned his back and started to walk away. When you gave up the obvious sugar and starch foods, the grim reaper realized that he might as well not even look back for you—not for a long while, at least.

When you began to give up the solid fats—butter, meat fat, all the dairy fats—he began to think of throwing in the towel. He knew that he was licked when you substituted the polyunsaturated for the hard, killer saturated fats. And premature death practically faded from view when you added ocean fish to your daily diet— vanquished by a sardine, a herring, the carriers of vanadium, zinc, the magic minerals. Say goodbye to death and hello to life.

Needless Fatalities from Heart Disease

The death rate from heart and blood vessel disease is high and is getting higher every year. This has been true for at least 30 years. How many of us stop and wonder *why* these figures are on the increase, *why* death from the number one killer is on the march? Surely, you would think, with all the tools and discoveries of modern science something might be done to halt these ravages. Something can be done, and you have already started to do it. In fact, the answer is so simple, so close to home, that most of us never see it. It is like Edgar Allen Poe's solution for hiding a letter. He left it right out in the open and it wasn't found! The answer to our problem of the number one killer is right out in the open. "Seek and ye shall find." "Knock and it shall be opened unto you." Turn the First Key to Longevity—the Key of Nutrition—and open the door to longer life.

Only You Can Do It

If there were a pill or potion to take, allowing us to continue to gorge ourselves on the killer foods, we would all take it. We are all lazy, looking for the easy way out, the magic wand, the magic pill, the magic formula. Well, there isn't any easier, safer, saner, more pleasant formula than the one I am showing you. There isn't any better way, free from side effects or complications, without drugs, without injections, without pain. There isn't any happier way, for I am showing you not only how to live a longer life, but also how to enjoy the added years. No pill or potion can do this for you.

Only *you* can do it. I am showing you the way, the Four Keys to Longevity, and you must pick them up and turn them, one after the other, in the door to long life and happiness. If you use these keys, you will become younger than you are now, slimmer and more attractive than you are now, healthier than you are now, happier than you are now, and, you will live a longer life.

Has Life Expectancy Really Increased?

Since 1900 medicine and surgery have made great strides. The antibiotics and sulfonamides have been developed, and many diseases that were formerly disabling or fatal have been conquered. Prevention of death in middle-age from such causes as pneumonia, tuberculosis, rheumatic heart disease, and many other infectious diseases, has increased life expectancy at birth by about 20 years. However—and here's the rub—life expectancy beyond the age of 50 has increased only 2.2 years. WHY? This is a big WHY! I think I can tell you why as follows.

Answer to the Big WHY of Life Expectancy

As you probably already have guessed, the answer to the big WHY is the increasing loss of our most active and productive men and women to coronary heart disease. This is the killer of the creative people, the benefit producers of our society. This is the grim reaper of the middle-aged and the elderly, and often of the young.

Everybody thinks that major advances in medical and surgical know-how have tremendously extended our human life-span. Actually, these advances have simply made it possible for children who would otherwise have died early in life to survive. That is the meaning of the statement that "life expectancy at birth for Americans has increased by about 20 years since 1900."

But since life expectancy beyond the age of 50 has increased only 2.2 years, we must conclude that there is actually *increased* mortality among those of middle years and beyond. This is obviously due to atherosclerotic coronary heart disease—our number one killer.

Life Expectancy Depends Greatly on Diet

It becomes more and more obvious to you, I am sure, that how long you or anyone else lives depends largely on what and how much you eat. The French have a saying that translates to tell us that "Death enters through the mouth." How sad to think that we dig our own graves every time we take that extra mouthful, that creamy-rich desert, that candy bar, that cream in our coffee, that mouth-watering steak.

How heart-breaking to realize that every time mother stuffs another mouthful into her beloved child, beaming at how roly-poly he is, she is preparing him for an early death. How tragic it is to think that the flower of our youth has already begun to develop the cholesterol deposits in their arteries that will make them statistics in the coronary death rate at an early age.

How doubly tragic when you and I know that *much of this could be prevented by simple changes in our eating habits.* By following the simple, painless and pleasant diet rules you have already learned *you* can put off the evil day, *you* can avoid becoming an early coronary statistic.

I know that you can do it because I have been proving it with my patients for well over 25 years. And I have proved it on myself as well!

My Own Case History of a Return from Death

I speak factually from long and sad personal experience. Let's start at the beginning and I will tell you my story, which I hope will benefit you in more than a few ways. Sit back in your consulting room chair, relax and listen.

Over 30 years ago I suffered from a disabling condition we doctors call "intermittent claudication." This is a very fancy name for spasm of the blood vessels of the legs. When the leg muscles began to feel the effect of the reduced blood flow through these spastic vessels, they became tight and painful. The calves of my legs became hard as rocks, the spasm of pain was intense, and I could not take another step.

Wherever I was at a spasm of pain, there I stopped. If it was in front of a window showing ladies lingerie, I looked at ladies lingerie. I could not move a step further until the spasm relaxed and the blood began to flow again through my blood vessels and into the spastic muscles. As time passed, it took longer and longer before I could move on.

At that time of my life I smoked cigarettes and a pipe. I really did not smoke very much, but since I knew the relationship between nicotine and the spasms I was suffering from, and as my condition became progressively worse, I gave up smoking. The blood vessel spasms became less and less, and within a relatively short time I could walk several blocks at a rapid pace before the claudication spasms returned. I had improved my condition a great deal by cutting out smoking, but I was far from cured.

The Doctor As A Patient

Some years later I became painfully aware of spasms of the arteries of still another region. I suffered an attack of the dreaded angina pectoris. This is a sharp, often disabling pain in the chest, usually in the heart region of the left chest. It is the result of a severe spasm of the coronary arteries, the vessels that bring blood to the heart muscle.

When the coronary arteries go into spasm, less blood reaches the heart muscle, and the blood-starved muscle cries out in pain. This is nature's warning signal—stop or die! Since this occurs with stress, with exercise, or after a heavy meal, the warning is clear—get rid of that stress! Stop that exercise! Eat less! I got the message. Since I was no longer smoking, the answer had to be found somewhere else.

While I was looking for the answer to my painful and possibly deadly problems, I had to find some way to control the pain. I refused to take drugs, and developed the pain control methods I later described in my book, *UNITROL: The Healing Magic of The Mind* (Parker Publishing Company, Inc.), but that is another story.

The answer to the basic problem was relatively simple. I was 60 pounds overweight—even according to the overly-liberal weight-height-age table of those days. I loved food, and was a gourmet who would drive 100 miles for a single dish I might have heard rumors about. I not only loved foods prepared with rich, creamy, fatty sauces, but I would eat large quantities. My choice was clear. I could either go on eating my way into an early grave, or I could reduce the size of my meals and the size of my waistline and live. It was either life or death, and since I still had much to do, many responsibilities, and many plans for the future, the killer calories and my deadly fat had to go.

The Doctor Treats Himself

Now began the research into the literature, long hours of study that culminated in an enormous bibliography of references in the world literature of science. The facts were there. I only needed to dig them out, arrange and rearrange them, and draw the proper conclusions. My motivation was sound and deep—*I wanted to live.*

I placed myself on a high protein diet while these studies were in progress. This allowed me to eat practically as much as I wanted while losing weight. Soon I found that the half-portion method was best. I did not miss the extra food. My stomach became smaller, since I was no longer distending it with enormous quantities of unnecessary food. When it reduced in size, it took less and less food to fill it; a full stomach gives us the signal that our appetite is satisfied, and it's no use to eat more.

As with practically everything else, moderation was the keynote. I ate in moderation and I ate the right foods to rid myself of the dangerous extra pounds. If you would like to see how I looked then —still too heavy after taking off many deadly pounds, go to the nearest medical library and look at a copy of my surgical textbook, *Ambulatory Proctology,* either the 1946 or the 1952 edition. On page 36 of the latter you will see the evidence. Now turn to the back cover of this book (the jacket) and see the "younger" present-day version of the same man, ten years later and many years younger!

How I Developed the Longevity Key—Nutrition

My studies resulted in the First Key to Longevity, the golden key of nutrition. Careful research convinced me that the answer to atherosclerotic heart disease was to be found in what we eat, in nutrition. I learned that this deadly disease was not merely a matter of calories, although this was certainly of basic importance to me since I was overweight.

Even more significant was the amount of fat in my diet. And still more important was the proportion of saturated to unsaturated fat. And that is how I finally evolved the polyunsaturated fat drink that has come to be known to my patients as the Cantor Cocktail. For me, and for those of my patients who are now living on it (quite literally), it has been a life-saving drink. Still later I learned about the magic minerals and the life-giving properties of ocean fish. And there is still more that I will tell you about as we continue our consultations—more that you can do to add years to your life.

My "Death" and "Rebirth"

During the time I was suffering from angina pectoris (pain in my heart region after exertion, stress, or a heavy meal) I consulted the best known cardiologist in New York. He made the diagnosis and suggested that I have a very special test of heart function. This test required that I go into a hospital and have an intravenous injection of an experimental drug, while heart tracings were being made (electrocardiograms).

I followed his advice and entered the hospital. The electrocardiograph wires were attached to my body in many locations, and the drug was then injected intravenously. My heart stopped a few minutes later.

The doctor had left the room (it was the cardiologist's assistant who was performing the test) and he did not return until after I had been "dead" for several minutes. As I learned later, he telephoned the chief, was told what to do in this desperate emergency, and I was restored to life.

As I returned to consciousness, every muscle in my body was in a state of fibrillation, vibrating like a taut violin string. I struggled back to awareness, *knowing that I had been dead*. Hours later my wife was telephoned by the hospital exchange and advised to come and get me. I had not told her that I was having this test, and the shock was enormous.

I decided to treat myself from that point on, and to avoid drugs unless it was a desperate emergency need.

This book, these consultations, are the fruits of my personal problems, my intensely personal need for an answer, and I hope that you will learn the lesson of life that they teach.

How to Be Intoxicated with Life

I learned many lessons from this difficult experience. One was to *avoid all drugs unless absolutely essential for the preservation of life.* I use many medications in the practice of medicine, but always with a specific indication and only well-tested drugs.

More important, I learned to be intoxicated with life. Life is a great dynamic gift. And yet we treat it lightly, take it for granted, and behave as though we were going to live forever. We ignore the banquet life spreads before us and see only a few crumbs. We thirst in the midst of the fountain of plenty, starve at a feast with plenty for all. I tell you now to allow yourself to be intoxicated with life. Be happy-drunk and not belligerent-drunk. See! Hear! Feel! Taste! Touch! Smell! Be aware of the little things, the sound of the wind in the trees, the feel of the rain in your face, the laughter of children. Be aware of the sad things—the tears of the unhappy, the tragedy of those who have lost a loved one, the hunger of the starving, the emptiness of the lonely, the depression of the failure, the terrible fear of the very sick and the dying—for these also make up life and must be experienced. Be intoxicated with life, see it all, accept it all, be grateful for it all—and try to be happy-drunk most of the time.

I will show you later on that we come this way many times, but only once in our present form. So enjoy every moment of your days, and your days and years will be well spent in creative awareness. Let your life be fun! All of it!

The Lesson of Diet and Life-Extension

I also learned the lesson of the vital diet factors for life-extension. The low calorie diet, the Cantor Cocktail, the magic minerals—

these were the key ingredients that made it possible for me to continue to cheat death to this point, well over 30 years. These simple nutritional principles of the First Key of Longevity will do the same for you.

Since atherosclerosis can be reversed and prevented, since overweight can be simply and pleasantly corrected, and since all this can be done without dangerous drugs or difficult diets, diseases of the heart and blood vessels can be reduced to a minimum. Always remember that the life you save may be your own. What I have done has been done by hundreds of my patients, and you can do the same.

Nutrition is the Major Key

Dr. Everett W. De Long was absolutely right when he said, "No chronic disease has ever found resolution *except through nutritional means.* Beri-beri, pernicious anemia, scurvy, pellagra, certain forms of heart disease, and polyneuritis are only a few of the once fatal chronic diseases that have found a resolution in nutritional science." And now you and I know that we can add atherosclerotic heart disease and atherosclerotic blood vessel disease to this list.

If you will follow all the instructions—the simple rules—that I will give you in these consultations, you will resolve your own chronic disease problems and you will be well on your way to the prevention of a cardiovascular death. If you do exactly as I say, you will rejoice in the realization of Dr. Edward Bortz that "We can throw away our canes, crutches and rocking chairs if we merely take advantage of what our doctors already know and try to tell us about how to live a century or more."

The Anti-Coronary Club

The Anti-Coronary Club, officially known as the Diet and Coronary Heart Disease Study Project, was started in New York in 1957 by the famed nutritionist, Dr. Norman Joliffe. Its purpose was to provide a public health test of the relationship between fats, diet, and health. The results of the study fully support the point of this book, that dietary control is a sound approach to the reduction of coronary heart disease. The results were as follows: In a famous study of coronary attacks in middle-aged people, conducted at

Framingham, Massachusetts, it was found that, on the average, there are 14.5 coronary attacks per 1,000 in the middle-aged group.

Now let's compare these figures with those of the Anti-Coronary Club group. The "members" of the Anti-Coronary Club, all of whom were on the low total fat and high polyunsaturated fat diet, had only 3.4 coronary attacks per 1,000! These figures are truly amazing, since they show the effect of a polyunsaturated fat diet on a large group.

This is further clinical proof of the value—the life-saving importance—of the rules for safe eating that I have been telling you about during our consultations. It is clinical proof, added to my own experience and the experience of many other researchers and nutritionists, that you can do a great deal to reduce your chance of ever suffering a coronary heart attack or a stroke.

More Life Through Less Cholesterol In Your System

What about the cholesterol level in the Anti-Coronary Club members? You will be happy to know that the diet the members were on lowered blood cholesterol levels in all cases! Those who initially showed the highest levels had the greatest reduction! So, once again you can quite literally "take heart." No matter how high your present blood cholesterol level may be, no matter what the present state of your heart and arteries, no matter what your age, the First Key of Longevity is for you. Use it and you will be helped.

After only six weeks of being on the special diet, the members of the Anti-Coronary Club had lowered their blood cholesterol levels and had reduced their chances for a fatal heart attack. That is what you can accomplish, and all you have to do is to start right now (if you haven't already begun your diet changes) on the life-saving, life-prolonging, low total fat, high polyunsaturated fat diet.

Let me translate that for you into the terms we have been using throughout these consultations, into the simple diet rules you already know. All this means is that you must eliminate the hard fats of meats and dairy products (this lowers the total fat you eat at the same time that it rids your diet of the saturated fats), and then drink the Cantor Cocktail three times a day (this gives you the polyunsaturated fats you need). That's all there is to it. That's all you need to do.

These studies prove that *as your diet goes, so goes your blood cholesterol level.* And as your cholesterol level goes, so goes your life. To lengthen life, to increase your years, you must decrease your blood cholesterol level. Fortunately, this is usually quite simple, and you already know exactly how to do it.

The American Heart Association Approves!

As a final note, let me add the words of the American Heart Association: "The reduction or control of fat consumption under medical supervision, with reasonable substitution of polyunsaturated for saturated fats, is recommended as a possible means of preventing atherosclerosis and decreasing the risk of heart attacks and strokes."

By now you can see the significance of this statement and even some of the reasoning behind it. You have seen some of the research behind it, and as we continue our discussions you will learn still more about keeping your body young and alive. You are as old as your arteries, and proper diet is your First Key to Longevity, the key that unlocks new flexibility, new youth for your arteries and for you.

More Tips for Happier Living While You Streamline Your Diet for Health

As I have so often said, there is little point in staying alive 100 or more years if you do not enjoy every one of them. And that is why I want to end each of our consultations with these tips for happier living.

1. Learn to live as if you were constantly in a condition of released inhibitions, or a total lack of them. Try to imagine yourself after a few drinks—very casual, carefree, happy. Be intoxicated with the simplicity of life, the beauty of little things, the pleasures of the moment.

2. You can't always win, and things will go wrong very often. When they do—stay calm. The tide will turn. All you have to do is to survive, to stay alive. Live long enough and all your enemies will have died, all your sorrows will have been relegated to the past. You will have outlived your troubles!

3. You only have to live life one day at a time. Certainly you can do that. Remember that life is made up of many battles. You will win some

and you will lose some. But if you stay alive long enough, you will have won your war.

And now for the best tip of all—you are immortal in health. You represent a chain of life that stretches back in unbroken continuity to the beginning of time, to the very first forms of life on this earth. I will prove this to you later on when we consider the Six Paths to Immortality (as I have proved it in my little book, *Immortality— Pathways to Peace of Mind.*) Since you are immortal—why worry?

Learn to accept this fact, and cheer yourself every time you are depressed by the way life is going, by telling yourself—over and over again—I AM IMMORTAL. I AM ETERNAL. I ALWAYS HAVE BEEN AND I ALWAYS WILL BE.

Besides, you are going to live long enough to outlive your sorrows, your lost battles, and all your enemies. You are learning how to live it up 100 or more years!

And NOW, in summary . . .

Once again we will review what you have learned to this point, so you can put your personal Longevity Program into prompt action. You must not delay. Start now, if you have not already begun, to restore youth to your aging tissues and organs, and vitality to every part of your body.

1. You must eat half-portions of what you used to eat, or even less.
2. You must cut out practically all starches and sugars.
3. You must not eat the animal fats or the dairy product fats.
4. You must substitute the polyunsaturated fats for these satrated animal and dairy fats.
5. You must drink your Cantor Cocktail before each meal.
6. You must eat ocean fish each day.
7. You must drink six to eight glasses of water each day (hard water if you can get it)
8. You may, if you wish, take a good vitamin-mineral product, recommended by your family physician, to give you the trace minerals that may be lacking in your water and food.

9. You have now learned how to say hello and goodbye to the number one killer—coronary heart disease.

10. You now know for an absolute proven fact that coronary heart disease may be avoided in several ways. Since this is so, you know—for an absolute fact—that your chances of living a long and healthy life are very very good if you follow the simple rules for eating that you have already learned.

11. You now know—for a fact, and from my own story of "death" and "rebirth"—that heart and artery disease can be conquered and that life can be greatly prolonged; that heart and artery disease can be reversed and the damaged heart and arteries can be restored to normal! I did it, and so can you!

12. You now have more tips for happier living, and you know how to live the life-happy, the intoxicated-with-life way (without alcohol!). Learn this and you will have added dynamic *life* to your years.

CHAPTER 5

HOW TO COPE WITH
THE CHOLESTEROL BULLET
THREATENING YOUR LIFE

Facts You Should Know About Fats in Your Body

You have learned the basic essentials of nutrition as they relate to prolonging life by improving or restoring the health of your heart and arteries. Obviously this is of enormous importance, since heart and artery disease will kill practically everybody who does not know and apply this knowledge.

During this consultation or chapter we will extend your knowledge of fats, tell you more about the "cholesterol bullet," and let you in on the meaning of hydrogenation—the meaning to your health. We will discuss animal versus vegetable fats, and I will instruct you on the mysteries of the body chemistry of fats. How your body works with fats will interest you, since this is closely tied in with the total fat-cholesterol problem. The more you know of the facts of life and the way your body works, the better able you will be to control your own nutrition. Knowledge is indeed power, and these chapter consultations will give you the knowledge you need to move swiftly and surely through the nutritional hazards of living.

We will consider the important question of, "How much cholesterol is normal?" Today's statistical normal equates with a high

49

level of statistical coronary deaths. There must be something wrong, and we will find out what that is and why.

You will also learn about the bonus offered by the high polyunsaturated fat diet—a bonus that gives you a slim, trim, new figure, radiantly healthy skin, and even eliminates spider varicosities of the legs in some cases.

And I will show you a startling fact—that your body can and does manufacture cholesterol from carbohydrates. That is why I have urged you to eliminate practically all carbohydrates from your diet as a first step in turning your Nutritional Key to Longevity when you unlock the door to longer and healthier life.

More Good News for Your Increased Longevity

I will tell you more about my Longevity Diet, adding some new food elements that you will enjoy. And I will tell you about a man who is 112 years old, and attributes his longevity to "fish." That doesn't surprise you, I know, but it is good to hear about those who have attained the goal you seek, the goal you too can reach if you will follow my advice.

And finally, we will talk about more tips for happier and better living. As I will tell you, again and again, there is little point in living 100 or more years if you are not enjoying life every happy step of the way. Life can be fun, and I hope to show you how to make it fun.

Are You Committing Suicide Unknowingly?

We are all committing suicide in one way or another, albeit in ignorance. If that seems like a startling statement, you may sit back and ponder over it for a moment. Relax in your consulting room chair and I will show you how practically everybody (if not everybody without exception!) is trying to kill himself, in one way or another.

Do you smoke? Our government has issued strong warnings through its health department to tell us that cigarette smoking is a major cause of cancer of the lung. If you are still smoking cigarettes, you are obviously trying to kill yourself.

Do you drink large amounts of alcohol? I am not against alcoholic beverages in moderation, but when you go beyond moderation you are heading for cirrhosis of your liver. Undoubtedly you know about the drinking man's diet, and the fact that the many versions of this diet to lose weight advocate taking alcohol with your meals. As a matter of fact, the more alcohol you take, the less apt you are to eat anything at all! Some stress-ridden business men simply "drink their lunch"; they are well on their way to chronic alcoholism, perhaps with cirrhosis of the liver.

How much alcohol is too much? Dr. Charles Lieber of Bellevue Medical Center, nationally known for his studies in alcoholic liver disease, believes that, "You don't have to be an underfed drunkard to have cirrhosis of the liver. Alcohol can damage the liver in the presence of a good diet. No matter how well one eats, if he drinks too much, he'll get a *fatty liver,* the advance warning of cirrhosis." Many seasoned travellers say that this is practically a status symbol in France. Dr. Lieber says that six to seven ounces per day of 86 proof whisky can be tolerated by the body, but "each person's level of tolerability is different."

As to the drinking man's diet, in my opinion those who follow any of these versions will feel that they have a license to drink, very much like James Bond's license to kill. This license to drink is a license to kill—to kill yourself! The followers of the martini-high-fat-diet are on their way to becoming skinny drunks with fatty livers and heart disease! Suicide? Absolutely!

Are you still eating full portions? Too many calories? Suicide? Certainly, and you know it!

Have you neglected to switch from the animal and dairy fats? Suicide? Tag! You're it!

Have you delayed drinking your Cantor Cocktail? Too much trouble to turn to page 165? Suicide? You know it is!

What about ocean fish each day? Not yet? Suicide by neglect? It sure is!

Are you drinking six to eight glasses of water each day? Not yet? Welcome to the slow suicide club.

I could go on and on, hour after hour, page after page, showing you the many ways in which you are committing suicide. Perhaps I should do just that, since you obviously cannot live out your natural life-span of 100 or more years if you commit suicide. But this should be enough to prove my point, and to show you once again that the helping hand you are looking for is at the end of your own arm, and it is this helping hand that will pick up or reject the wrong foods, the wrong drinks, and so on. *You* must make the decision for yourself. What will it be—life or death?

The Slow but Deadly Cholesterol Bullet

We have been talking about suicide, suicide with "slow" bullets. Regardless of whether the bullet is slow or sudden, the vital organ is pierced just as surely, and death is just as inevitable. Cholesterol is one of the slow bullets, often fired in earliest youth, only to reach its mark years later, piercing an artery of the heart or the brain. This type of suicide is perhaps murder when it begins in childhood. When mother stuffs her youngster with food—especially candy and ice cream—in the sadly mistaken notion that being fat is evidence of good health, she is firing the slow cholesterol bullet herself. She would not do it if she knew the facts, and she must be forgiven for her tragic lack of knowledge. But the damage will be done, whether she means to do it or not.

To really understand cholesterol you need to know something about fats in general. I will tell you a little about the structure of fats, since cholesterol is one of the "simple fats." Actually, *fats* and *oils* mean the same thing, the only difference being that fats are solid at room temperature, while oils are liquid at the same temperatures. Those fats which have a low melting point—the ones that are usually liquid—ordinarily have a larger proportion of unsaturated fatty acids than do the solid fats. This gives you a most important indicator—a way to tell which fats are the "killer fats." As you now know, the solid fats are the deadly ones.

What You Should Know About the Chemistry of "Lipids"

You will read about *lipids* in the semi-technical literature, in the well-written science columns of the major newspapers, and so forth. Fats and oils belong to the larger class of foods known as *lipids*. You will recognize a lipid by the fact that it will not dissolve in water, but will dissolve in such fat solvents as ether, carbon tetra-chloride, benzene, or acetone. Since none of these solvents are found in the body, and since most of them are, in fact, deadly poisons when taken by mouth, it is obvious that lipids will not be dissolved and will stay in your body to a very large extent. This is an over-simplification, of course, but it will do to emphasize the fact that cholesterol—a waxy fat—can and does line the interior of your vital coronary arteries, since there is nothing in your blood to dissolve it and to wash it away.

Once deposited, this deadly waxy-fat will not be removed by the blood if there is already a high level of cholesterol in your blood stream. Now you begin to see the importance of lowering the level of your blood cholesterol by the "magic" of diet, the First Key to Longevity.

The Dangers of Hydrogenation of Food to Your Blood Stream

If you read the labels on margarine, or listen to the radio and television advertising, or read the science writers, you have heard about hydrogenation. Hydrogenation is the process used commercially to convert liquid fats into solids. In this process the liquid fats are subjected to a high temperature in the presence of hydrogen gas. This converts the oils, which would be liquid at ordinary room temperatures, to fats which are solid, *saturated,* and dangerous for your vital blood vessel life-lines.

Hydrogenated, then, simply means hydrogen has been added. The liquid fats are saturated with hydrogen, for it is the amount of hydrogen in the fat that determines whether it is liquid or solid, un-saturated or saturated, safe or dangerous. Now you will understand that polyunsaturated simply means that there is even less hydrogen in the fatty *oil* or in the margarine or in the fish, etcetera. Curious, isn't it, to think that from the point of view of the chemist, it is hydrogen—a gas—that determines how long you and I will live? Still more curious, perhaps, when you realize that traces of minerals such as vanadium, zinc, and magnesium also play their part in our personal drama of life and death. Less curious, though, when you realize that we are little more than an accumulation of inorganic and organic chemicals, largely seawater, put together to generate electricity within our battery-like cells.

If you think this is far-fetched, stop for a moment and realize that your heart gives off electrical currents, originating in a little bundle of tissue called the pacemaker, that determines your heart rate and its regularity. The electrocardiogram measures these waves, these electrical currents. And beyond that is the fact that the amount of certain trace minerals in your bloodstream control this vital pacemaker.

Your brain gives off electrical currents that are measurable with the electroencephalogram—very much like the electrocardiogram. The chemistry of your blood controls this also, to some degree. There is no doubt that electrical tracings could be made from any and all parts of the human body. Some day they will be, and such tracings for the kidneys, the liver, and so forth, will be just as commonly used as the heart and brain wave tracings are today.

Keep Your Energy Dynamos Working for Longer Life

Dr. Selye, the famed Montreal researcher you already have met, believes that each person has only a limited amount of energy in his energy bank, and when he has made the last withdrawal, life comes to an end. He believes that stress, the anxieties and problems and pressures of everyday living, draw heavily upon our energy bank.

If this is true, you must conserve your energies, avoid stress, and live simply if you want to live longer.

But I suspect that our energies, although not unlimited certainly, can be restored regularly, just as a nickel-cadmium battery can be recharged when it runs low. In my opinion, you will revitalize your electric energies, your cellular capacity, when you change your diet to the longevity pattern already partially described for you. Certainly the trace minerals are essential for proper energy production. So are vitamins. And so are the polyunsaturated fats, high grade proteins such as those in ocean fish, and the small amount of carbohydrate and starch that you cannot avoid in any well-balanced diet. *Your best bet for keeping your energy dynamos functioning at capacity is to eat properly.*

Circulation is the Key to Tissue Function

Every cell of your body requires a good blood flow to bring it the proper nutrients so that it can function to best advantage. This means that your arteries must be kept open and flexible. And that, in turn, means that you must get rid of anything clogging or obstructing those arteries. Cholesterol is the common obstruction, and the Longevity Diet will clean out your arteries. Since proper cell function is essential for good tissue and organ function, it is equally obvious that you must keep the life-lines of your arteries open and operating at capacity. This is the way you maintain the best possible flow of electrical energy throughout your body. This is the way you keep your home energy dynamos in good repair.

In my opinion, as long as your energy dynamos are in good repair you stand a good chance of living 100 or more years. You can't overdraw your energy bank as long as you keep a healthy balance in your account. The Longevity Diet provides the internal "energy deposits" that your body translates into nutrients for an unobstructed blood stream, nutrients that your body converts to stored energy as well as to current energy for your daily needs.

Fats—Their Effect on Life Functions

And now we are ready to talk about digestion and absorption of fats—what your body does to the fats you eat as they move along through your stomach and intestinal tract. *First, no fat is digested in the mouth.* Fat is broken down into its components to some extent in the stomach by a digestive enzyme of the pancreas. But here is a most important point to remember: the length of time the food remains in your stomach depends upon the amount of fat in your stomach. I have already told you the importance of this when I discussed the Cantor Cocktail. You will recall that one of the great advantages of this cocktail is the fact that it acts as a natural appetite depressant, due to its fat content. The fat slows the emptying time of the stomach, and keeps the stomach filled—even with a relatively small amount of food compared to the amount you would eat if it kept pouring out of your stomach as fast as you ate it. Another advantage of the special polyunsaturated fat cocktail is that it depresses appetite in one other way. Fat has a high satiety value, which means that fat satisfies the appetite best, better than protein, starch or sugar. So, if you will take your Cocktail before each meal, as directed, *you will want less food and you will need less food.*

In your small intestine, the pancreatic enzyme breaks down fats so that they can be absorbed into your blood stream. In that way the digestion and absorption of fats is complete before your large intestine is reached by the food you eat.

Animal Fats Versus Vegetable Fats

You already know the important fact of the battle between animal and vegetable fats—the fact that eminent medical researchers have observed an increase in blood cholesterol when you take large amounts of fats in your diet. This increase in the level of the deadly cholesterol bullet is greatest when you take large amounts of the hard animal and dairy fats. It is lowest when you substitute the polyunsaturated vegetable oils for the animal and dairy saturated fats. These facts give you the key to one of the first principles of your new Longevity Diet. You must cut down the total amount of fat in your foods—*even the polyunsaturated fats,* and you must try to eliminate the saturated animal and dairy fats as much as possible.

I would advise that you buy your oils in a health food store, since they are cold pressed and have no additives (chemical preservatives). If there is no health food store in your town, however, you can use the products in your local grocery or supermarket. My recommendation is merely an added margin of safety based upon my dislike for chemical additives, and my personal preference for pure, unadulterated products.

How Much Cholesterol Is Normal?

It is my carefully considered opinion, based upon many years of medical practice and study, that the cholesterol level that passes for "normal" in our country is much too high. Most laboratories use the figures of 150 to 250 mg. per 100 cc. of blood as the normal level when reporting to physicians. But, as I have repeatedly said, it is also considered "normal" for most of us to die quite young, and equally "normal" for our death to be due to coronary or other blood vessel disease. I disagree, and heartily so!

Statistics on blood cholesterol levels in countries where death from heart and blood vessel disease is relatively uncommon (compared to the United States), show much lower levels than ours. The "normal" level in those countries is about 150 mg. per 100 cc. of blood, and not higher. I believe that this is the proper level for everyone, regardless of where he or she lives. I believe that this is the level *you* should try for. Your best chance of succeeding in your search for longer life and renewed youth is offered by the First Key to Longevity, the golden Key of Nutrition. Cut your food intake to the minimum required by your type of work, replace saturated by unsaturated fats, add ocean fish to your daily diet, drink six to eight glasses of hard water each day, and follow all the other rules you are about to learn.

You Have the Power of Life and Death

If the cholesterol bullets are to be kept out of your arteries, and especially out of your coronary arteries and the arteries of the brain, they must first be kept out of your blood stream. Always remember that it is your blood stream which carries the cholesterol bullets to your heart and brain, and that it is your mouth that receives the deadly fats, sugars, and starches that are converted into the ultimate cholesterol bullets. *You* are the one who is responsible. *You* are the one who puts food into your own mouth. *You* are the one who must decide your own destiny.

Cholesterol Case History of a Middle-Aged Housewife,

This patient was a 47-year old housewife who had been brought up to believe that she committed a sin if she did not eat every morsel of food on her plate. Her three brothers and one sister had been given the same belief, and they all were enormously overweight. She was 56 pounds overweight—short, fat and ungainly. She needed help for many conditions resulting from her excess pounds. She had a colon problem, with overactivity and excess mucus secretion, high blood pressure, and diabetes in its early stage. In addition, she was emotionally disturbed by the pressures of trying to make ends meet, even as you and I.

She wanted her large bowel condition cleared up, but refused to do anything about her excess weight, her hypertension, and diabetes, since these conditions required that she restrict her diet as a fundamental first step. I told her that she was committing suicide, but she refused to listen. *Her mother's early teaching, consciously or subconsciously, stayed with her and took precedence over anything I might say.*

Her bowel condition (mucous colitis) cleared up quite well with appropriate treatment (see *Ridding Yourself of Psychosomatic Health Wreckers* if you are interested in details in such cases), but she died at 52 years of age. The cause of death? Stroke! Suicide? Yes. The underlying cause? Mother's well-meaning but deadly misinformation that "you must clean your plate and leave nothing." Okay if you are eating half-portions, but potentially deadly if you are eating mother-size portions. Do you want to be a suicide?

Added Benefits of the Low Fat Diet

Since the fats deposited in your body tissues are extremely sensitive to unsaturated fats reaching them through your blood stream, when you reduce the amount of saturated animal fats in your diet and increase the amount of unsaturated vegetable fats, you deposit soft (and safe) fat as a *replacement* for much of your present hard fat deposits. Is that a long and complicated sentence? Okay, let's translate for simplicity.

Your present body fats are the hard type, just like all other animal fats. If you continue to eat more hard (animal) fats, your body fat stays hard. But if you substitute the polyunsaturated vegetable fats for the hard fats in your diet, your body fat soon changes to the soft type. You get rid of the hard fats in your tissues, and you replace them by soft fats. Naturally, for you are what you eat! This is particularly true if you are on a low carbohydrate diet at the same time. You see, carbohydrates are also converted into hard fats by our bodies.

Once again we can safely say that when you have been on the Longevity Diet for a relatively short time, you will have replaced large amounts of your present hard fat deposits by the softer, unsaturated fatty acids.

If you are now overweight, and want to reduce, this soft fat allows your skin to better mould itself to your new sleek contours. You will become slimmer, but not baggy-skinned and older looking. How is that for a bonus of the Longevity Diet?

There is another bonus. In my clinical experience I have observed that patients on the high polyunsaturated fat diet develop softer, smoother, almost satin-like skin.

And I have still another bonus to offer as to *gaining weight*. One of my male patients, who elected not to kill himself, also observed that the many "spidery" looking varicose veins in the skin of his lower legs disappeared after only a few months on the Longevity Diet. He was not overweight, incidentally, but rather slim—a sixty-five-year old, very tired and worn-out mechanic. He *gained weight* on the Longevity Diet, coming very close to the designated age-height weight table requirement. His blood cholesterol of 350+ returned gradually to 250, then to 200+, and finally to 165. His hardened arteries (which I could feel in his arms) became softer, and he became more vigorous and active than he had been in years.

These are what I call the clinical bonuses of the First Key to Longevity. They are bonuses that add much to your goal of revitalization of tissues and prolongation of life.

The Cholesterol Bullet Is Aimed Not Only at Your Arteries

Your arteries are not the only cholesterol bullet targets. These are obviously the most dangerous, the most vital target areas, but the cholesterol bullets reach other parts of the body as well. For example, abnormal fatty deposits may ruin your liver, especially if your diet is high in saturated fats. There may even be an accumulation of cholesterol in the liver when there is a deficiency of essential fatty acids in your diet.

There are other diseases in which cholesterol bullets reach unusual body locations. These diseases are called atheromatoses. If you have such a problem, there will be fatty deposits in your eyelids and on tendons, as well as in your blood vessels. Sometimes there are also fatty deposits in the heart lining itself. I would suggest that you look at your eyelids right now, and if you see yellow nodules, let your doctor check your general condition and your blood cholesterol level. For that matter, it is always safest to have a careful general examination before starting on any diet or other health regimen.

Your Body Manufactures Cholesterol

It may seem strange that your body manufactures cholesterol normally. Every person manufactures cholesterol, since cholesterol is a normal ingredient of important body tissues, hormones, and so forth. It is only when your body manufactures an excessive amount that trouble occurs. And, of course, if you add to the natural self-produced cholesterol a large additional food supply of solid fats, you may well be in for trouble.

By some strange chemistry, not even fully understood by medical researchers, *your body can convert protein to carbohydrate* (and this is what happens to 58 per cent of the protein you eat!), and this carbohydrate in turn may go on to become cholesterol!! This should convince you, if nothing else does, of the importance of half-portions, limiting your calories, and even limiting the essential protein foods.

Since almost anything you eat becomes a possible source of cholesterol bullets, the less you eat the better it is for your heart, arteries and liver.

112 Years Old and Still Young

When we began our consultation today I promised to tell you about a man who lived to be 112, and was still going strong. Ocean fish is the answer (or at least part of the answer), and this comes as no surprise to you since you are now well aware of the almost magical properties of ocean fish. You know of the polyunsaturated fats in such fish, and of the vanadium and zinc. You also know that fish provides a very excellent protein—and it is protein that furnishes the amino acid building blocks for all your tissues' growth and repair.

The *New York Times* reported the 112th birthday of a Japanese fisherman. When asked to what he attributed his longevity, he replied with the single magical word—"fish." Little more need be said except that the diet of the fisherman is all too often what most people would consider minimal in terms of the amount of calories consumed. We can probably assume that this 112-year-old fisherman owed his long and active life to the combination of a fish diet and a low caloric diet. That is the ideal combination for you.

When I go to fish restaurants in New York and other cities, I like to order the fish stew of the French fishermen—a peasant staple called bouillabaise. This simple fish stew-soup combination contains all the ingredients you might wish for a tasty and healthful dish—it is made with whatever fish is in season, for the most part. But it is quite expensive in the sea food restaurant, even though it is the staple soup-stew dish of the Fresh peasant, and quite inexpensive for them. You can make it at home for relatively little, and you should try it soon.

I think you will like it.

More Tips for Better Living and Its Enjoyment

As with each of our consultation sessions, I want to conclude this one by giving you a few more tips on how to enjoy your new-found health and your added years.

1. "There is no duty we underrate so much," wrote Robert Louis Stevenson, "as the duty of being happy." Like Stevenson, I would suggest that you find your own happiness by helping others to be happy.

Stevenson spent the last few years of his life in Samoa, and when one of the chiefs was imprisoned by a European government, Stevenson visited him regularly. He brought him tobacco and other gifts. When the chief was released, he and other chiefs built a road through the wilderness to Stevenson's house, and they did it with their own hands. They called the road the "Road of Gratitude." When Stevenson died at 44 (he was a life-long invalid), the natives he had befriended buried him on a mountain top. So that the birds would sing undisturbed over his grave, they forbade the use of firearms on that mountain forever.

And so I bid you be happy. And I bid you seek your happiness in helping others. Bring happiness to others and you will bring happiness to yourself.

2. Try to make a new friend every day, but most of all, try to keep your old friendships in good repair. New friends are silver, but old friends are gold. Woodrow Wilson told us, and I agree, that, "Friendship is the only cement that will hold the world together."

3. When things are going right, let yourself enjoy life. Tell yourself that all is well, and *allow yourself to feel happy*. Too often we get set in a gloom habit, and forget how to smile—even when things are going right.

4. Stop thinking negatively. Give yourself a break and tell yourself, "I am feeling better and better, happier and hapier." You will be surprised to find that this will give you a lift, even during rough times.

And NOW, in summary...

Before you leave my consulting room, I want to review the important features of this consultation.

1. You know the basic essentials of nutrition as they relate to prolonging life by improving the health of your heart and arteries.
2. You have considered the question of whether or not you are trying to commit suicide—and what to do about it.
3. You have learned the many hidden ways in which we are all trying to commit suicide, and all about the various "slow bullets."
4. You have learned the truth about the various forms of drinking man's diet, and the truth about alcohol.
5. You now have the facts on the cholesterol bullet.
6. You now know that the cholesterol "bullet" is often fired first in infancy and childhood, with the very best intentions —often by our own mother!
7. You now know the chemistry of fats and the difference between fats and oils, both in the lipids class. In simple language, you have learned *why* the polyunsaturated fats are best for you, and *why* the hard fats are dangerous.
8. You have learned what *hydrogenation* means, and how to avoid the hydrogenated fats.
9. You have learned how to keep your body dynamos in the best possible condition—how to recharge your batteries.
10. You have learned that circulation is the key to good tissue function, and what you must do to improve your own circulation.
11. You have learned what happens to fats when they enter your intestinal tract.
12. You have learned more about animal versus vegetable fats, and what this means to your own heart and arteries.
13. You have learned about the different types of polyunsaturated oils available in the stores, and which you should buy.
14. You now know how much cholesterol is normal—knowl-

edge that may tilt the balance between life and death for you.

15. You have read case histories that show you how the final answer is in your own hands. You yourself can now determine whether you will live or die.

16. You have learned the added bonuses from the low fat diet, bonuses that will give you a healthier liver, a clearer, younger skin, and a more youthful figure and face. You may even get rid of spider varicosities on your legs.

17. You have learned how your body manufactures cholesterol, and what this means to you.

18. You have also learned a few more tips on how to *live* a happier and more productive life.

CHAPTER 6

HOW TO USE
THE LIFE-SAVING
"DEFENDER FATS"

We will begin by reviewing briefly the information you have already put into action in revising your daily diet to prolong and revitalize your life.

1. You are eating half portions or less, in order to reduce your total calories.

2. You have substituted the polyunsaturated vegetable fats, especially safflower oil, for the animal and dairy hard fats.

3. You are drinking the Cantor Cocktail each day, before each meal.

4. You are eating ocean fish at least once a day.

5. You are drinking several glasses (at least seven or eight, I hope) of hard water each day. If you can't get hard water, you are taking a daily mineral-vitamin tablet or capsule prescribed by your family physician.

6. You have eliminated all possible starches and sugars from your diet, realizing that these provide both empty calories and still more cholesterol as they are taken into your system.

7. You are already becoming slimmer, trimmer, and feel better than you have in years.

8. You are learning to enjoy life, to live it one day at a time, and to really feel, see, hear, taste and touch every thrilling moment.

During this consultation I will tell you more about the life-saving defender fats. I will give you some facts on what a calorie means, and how many you need, based on your sex, age, weight, height and occupation.

I will have some special instructions for those of you who are overweight, and will tell you why you must avoid rapid weight gains. A little later on, during another series of special consultations that I have called The Second Key to Longevity, I will teach you all you need to know in order to lose weight without drugs, *even while you sleep!*

I will have something to say about the moderate "slip" in eating habits, and will show you that *you need never feel imprisoned by this or any other diet.* You and I are human, and are therefore entitled to act in a human fashion—to slip up once in awhile and indulge ourselves. We will talk about that later on during this consultation.

Then I will tell you how the defender fats do their protective job to save you from the deadly killer fats. They work in mysterious ways, and you will enjoy learning their mysteries.

I will tell you about the American Killer Breakfast, and how substitution is the key to longer life, in addition to moderation. I will teach you many other important life-saving facts as we talk together, and I will end this consultation—as I have all the others—with more tips for happier living while living longer.

Killer Fats Versus Defender Fats

You know that the saturated fats are the culprits in atherosclerosis and coronary heart disease. Clinical studies, experimental laboratory findings, and all other evidence supports this point. You know also that a high blood cholesterol level is associated with most cases of atherosclerosis. You have seen that the lower your blood cholesterol level is, the healthier you will probably be and the longer you will probably live.

Finally—and perhaps most important—you have been shown how your blood cholesterol level can be altered relatively rapidly *by simple diet changes,* and how such diet changes will help you rid your vital arteries of their present cholesterol deposits. This is the secret of the polyunsaturated fats versus the saturated fats. This is the secret you now know and—I hope—have already put into action to conserve and prolong your own life.

Special Instructions if You Are Overweight

For those of you who are overweight, I have a few special instructions to help you understand why and how you must rid yourself of those excess pounds. First turn to the table of normal weight-height-age levels (page 144) and check your statistics against the proper weight level for your own sex, age and height. If you are now overweight, it is urgent that you reduce to the safe level as soon as possible.

I do not mean that you are to go on a crash diet, a fad diet, a mono diet, or any starvation routines. Under medical supervision any of the unusual diet or starvation methods may be quite safe, but if you are going it alone, *avoid such crash programs.* You need not lose more than one to three pounds each week. If you have already begun to follow my Longevity Diet instructions—half portions, and so on—you have probably already lost several of those unsightly and unhealthy pounds. Simply eliminating the carbohydrates and starches (the real key to the so-called drinking man's diet variations) will turn the trick for you. The combination of the half-portion idea with the low sugar and starch approach and the three ounces of safflower oil in your daily Cantor Cocktails, offers an unbeatable weight-losing approach. You will not need any drugs to suppress your appetite, since this diet is quite filling, denies you nothing of value, and even provides the natural appetite-depressant action of the safflower oil fats. But I again repeat, as I do in all my books, it would be desirable to see your family physician before going on any diet. Although you are here now in my "consulting room," and I am happy to give you any advice and help you may need, you also need to have a general examination by your family doctor, a study of your blood cholesterol level, blood sugar, and so on, and also a protein-bound iodine blood test to show the level of activity of your thyroid gland.

Why Simple Blood Tests Are Desirable for Diet Control

Simple tests of your metabolism, your blood fat level, and so on, only require a single specimen of blood from an arm vein. They can all be done with one vein puncture (a quick, inexpensive, almost painless office procedure).

For the study of your thyroid function, I prefer the blood test for protein-bound iodine to the more expensive and less accurate breathing metabolism test. I will have much more to say about this when we get to the Second Key for Longevity in this book.

Now the fact of the matter is that most of you will be able to lose those deadly extra pounds *without any drugs.* The Longevity Diet does the work for you even while you are enjoying gourmet food, perhaps ocean fish in Bouillabaisse style, or broiled or fried in safflower oil, and many other foods you now enjoy. You will not go hungry, and the simple "restrictions" are only against the denatured foods of our so-called civilization (sugars, starches). But if you do need help, it may only be the tiny thyroid analog pills that contain the active principle of the thyroid gland. This will perk up your metabolism and send you happily along the road to your new, slim, trim, supple, youthful figure and face.

Lower Your Weight and Your Blood Cholesterol Falls

When you lose the unsightly and dangerous extra pounds, your blood cholesterol will also be lowered in practically every case. This is because you have eliminated the saturated fats (the killer fats), and have substituted the defender fats (the polyunsaturated fats). It is also because you have eliminated most of the starch and sugar from your diet as prescribed in the Longevity Diet.

In my experience, the blood cholesterol level falls rather regularly during the early weeks of weight reduction, assuming you are losing weight sensibly by means of the Longevity Diet. And best of all, it will stay low as long as you remain on your low total fat, polyunsaturated oil diet.

Why You Must Avoid Rapid Weight Gain

In a careful study of obesity, fat metabolism, and cardiovascular disease, it was discovered that simple overeating with rapid weight gain will lead to a marked increase in the cholesterol serum—obviously very dangerous to our goal of longevity. What does this mean to you who are now overweight from overeating? The damage is already done, but as you know from this book, it is reversible. The cholesterol in your blood and in your arteries can be removed or altered. Your arteries can be made more flexible again.

But here is the important lesson, the warning of this experiment. Since you are now overweight and reducing, you must never slip back into your consistently bad former habit of overeating. If and when you do, your blood cholesterol level will go even higher than it was before you lost weight! Ponder that for a sober moment!

Once you have begun your Longevity Diet, once you have decided that you really want to stay alive and vigorous as long as possible, you must stay on it for obvious reasons.

A Case History of a Housewife's Falling Off the Longevity Diet

Let's take a look at the record of a patient of mine. She is a housewife with high blood pressure, constantly tired and anxious, and more than *60 pounds overweight*. She is only 34 years of age. Her laboratory record showed a high blood cholesterol level of 350+ per 100 cc of blood during the first three months of my "treatment." Why? She claimed that she was following the Longevity Diet, but when I asked her to bring me a record of every food she ate during a single week's time, the fact was that she was eating cake, sugar-filled coffee, and other forbidden foods, especially ice cream, whenever she felt tired while shopping. "I need it to keep me going," was her plaintive protest. The fact of the matter was that if she didn't take anything but water, vitamins, and minerals for a week or more, she would have had no difficulty in "keeping going" full steam ahead!

She did follow the Longevity Diet faithfully after that, and her blood cholesterol level came down to 250 rather rapidly, and then to 210, and still later to 160±. That was very good indeed, and she was grateful for the new vitality, the new energy, and the new figure, for she had lost her excess weight at the same time.

Six months later I saw her again, this time for a truly disabling constipation problem. I was dismayed by her return to her "fortress of fat," and still more distressed by her blood cholesterol level. It was now well over 400! Her blood pressure was also back in the stratosphere. She had emotional problems that were driving her to constant eating—literally to the slow bullets of food "suicide."

The Lessons for You from This Housewife's Case History

If you are now overweight and reducing, these are the lessons you must learn from the case of the housewife I have described. See your doctor to be sure that you don't also have other problems such as high blood pressure, diabetes, or arthritis, for these often occur with obesity.

If you have emotional problems that are driving you to commit "suicide" by overeating, you must find out what they are and get rid of them. I have described exactly how you can do this yourself in two other books—*UNITROL: The Healing Magic of The Mind,* and *Ridding Yourself of Psychosomatic Health Wreckers.* In all fairness to yourself, if this is your present problem, you should read these two books and get rid of the underlying emotional dynamite that is driving you to food suicide.*

You Can "Slip" in Your Diet Program Once in a While

I don't want to leave you with the impression that you are imprisoned by the rules of the diet as you would be by the bars of a jail cell. You may shudder at the thought of *never* indulging an occasional craving for sugar, something sweet, or even a fatty, juicy piece of rare steak. After all, even though your life may be at stake, it is not always easy to abruptly and completely give up the habits of a lifetime. We are all human, and being human means that we all make mistakes—often over and over again. Freud was right when he spoke of the "repetition compulsion" that drives each of us to repeat the same mistakes over and over again. The main idea is to control impulses intelligently.

It is often extremely difficult for many of my patients to pass up the "gooey" deserts and saturated fat foods to which they have habituated themselves since childhood. I do not ask you to do it, believe it or not. I do not expect you to be "good" all the time. No one can.

I expect you to make the "moderate slip" from time to time, especially during the early days and weeks of your diet. I still do, occasionally, so why shouldn't you!

---

* Full information is available from the UNITROL Teaching Institute, 147-41 Sanford Ave., Flushing, N.Y. 11355.

Subconscious and Conscious Resistances to Diet Programs

There are both subconscious and conscious resistances to eliminating candies and cakes. Candy was a reward for being good, a reward you were trained to expect from childhood on. When you "grew up" you continued to give yourself this "reward," either for accomplishment or for solace when "things went wrong." You probably still have this early training habit of taking sweets when things go wrong. Most of us do, so don't feel too badly about it. That is why, if you try to force yourself to stay very strictly within the regulations of the Longevity Diet, you will be building up all sorts of resistances in your subconscious mind.

When your subconscious mind becomes resistant (when logic encounters the emotions, the emotions always win), you will suddenly discover all kinds of "reasons" for breaking the rules. This is called rationalization. You try to find rational reasons for emotional behavior. Remember that it is your subconscious that has the final word in guiding all behavior, and that your early and now-forgotten training and emotions will emerge victorious if you don't watch out. This early training provides many of the slow bullets, fired constantly by your mind and mine, triggering our dangerous eating habits and other forms of suicide. I will tell you more about what to do to guard yourself against your own subconscious mind in later consultations. For the moment you need only be aware of the problem, and recognize it when it occurs. Don't succumb by giving up your Longevity Diet, or you will be a suicide and a premature mortality statistic.

Obviously, this is why I advocate yielding to the occasional urge with a moderate "slip." Give in a little to avoid giving in completely. Bend or you will break.

How To Keep Your Subconscious Happy During a Diet Program

To keep your subconscious happy until you learn how to replace your previous and present patterns of action with health-giving and affirmative new patterns of behavior, take an occasional candy or cake "reward." Indulge yourself from time to time, if the urge is overpowering. As time goes by, as you see yourself becoming younger, slimmer, healthier, and as your subconscious further absorbs the principles I am teaching you, these "cravings" for fat, sugar, and cholesterol bullet types of foods will disappear, for you will have newer and better incentives to stay on the Longevity Diet.

Be Human and Be Happy Makes Sense in Diet Matters

One of the main reasons why I will permit you to "slip" from time to time is simply because we must recognize human nature for what it is. Like any new experience, the Longevity Diet must be learned, must be "tried out," and until the time that it becomes fully entrenched in your daily life, you may "slip" from time to time. You do it with my full understanding and *temporary approval* —as long as you stay within the limits of the "moderate slip." Don't overdo it or you will lose the full benefits of the Longevity Diet.

How to Rationalize in Rejecting Harmful Foods

Do not feel guilty about it, and do not become discouraged. Simply go on, and try to limit the number of "slips." You will have little trouble doing this if you look at the sugar-heavy, fat-saturated, cholesterol bullet foods in terms of their high caloric content and their saturated fat levels. Instead of seeing an ice cream sundae, a slice of bacon, or a piece of strawberry shortcake as things that are "good" (meaning simply that they have tasted "good" to you in the past), look at them as foods that are drenched with fat and death-dealing cholesterol. See them as unsightly and heart-destroying extra pounds of weight. When you look at such foods, see them as enemies of your heart and arteries. Think of what happens to your heart and arteries, the cholesterol deposits that threaten your very existence, each time you succumb to the tempting cake, candy, pie, and other cholesterol bullets.

In short, think of your life, and how much *life-time* you surrender each time you indulge in a few brief moments of pleasant taste sensation. It isn't worth the price, I know—and given time, you too will agree.

Nevertheless, I do not want you to feel guilty over an occasional "fall from grace." I only ask that you consider the price your heart and arteries must pay, and try to limit your "slips" as time goes by.

How A Taxi Driver Beat His Health Problem with the Longevity Diet

A taxi driver, upon whom I had operated for hemorrhoids (using my ambulatory office method), asked me for help in overcoming the excess pounds he had accumulated from "sitting all day" (a very common complaint) followed by his wife's excellent and very abundant meals (which relaxed him) when he finished his day's work. Although only 46 years of age then, he looked 20 years older.

I put this patient on the Longevity Diet to help him get rid of his extra pounds and to restore some measure of vitality to his tissues. He did lose weight gradually, but his blood cholesterol level kept shooting back to the high levels of the past. His problem originated from the fact that he stopped at frequent intervals throughout his working day to pick up and eat one or two candy bars at a time.

I pointed out that he was asking for serious trouble by doing this. Each time that he allowed his blood cholesterol level to go back up *it tended to return to higher and higher levels.* This posed a serious threat to his heart and his vital arteries, and I told him the facts about that.

He understood and changed his habits as prescribed in this book. I did not see him again for a while. When he entered my consulting room I did not recognize him. He looked no more than in his late thirties, and he had the bounce and vitality of a very young man, although his age was then 56. He explained this tremendous health dividend as follows:

Both he and his wife had adopted the Longevity Diet pattern of eating and living, and both had become literally new, healthier, younger people. His cholesterol level was now 155 mg. per 100 cc of blood and he no longer endangered himself by the candy-bar "slips." *You* can do the same by keeping your own "slips," your own lapses into the twilight zone of sugars, starches and fats, to an absolute minimum.

How the Defender Fats Guard Your Health

As you know, the "defender" fats are the polyunsaturated fats. The ones I recommend for you are safflower oil, corn oil, and the very unsaturated fats of fish. So we must look to the vegetables and the oceans for our defense against the number one killer and his number one henchman—the saturated killer fats.

I am not specially recommending vegetarianism to you, although it offers an excellent way of nutritional life. Man is a hunter by nature, and therefore a meat and fish eater. But those vegetarians who eat only fruits, nuts and vegetables have definitely lower cholesterol levels than those who eat meat. As I have commented before, it is almost as though man is being punished as a killer when he kills and eats animals only to have the very animals he eats kill him in turn! But this is only poetic fancy, since it is the way of nature that all forms of life, large or small, feed upon other forms of life. For that matter, vegetables are very much alive, and undoubtedly have some "feelings," although not in human terms.

I want to make it very clear, then, that far from demanding vegetarianism, my Longevity Diet allows you a very wide range of foods, all of which are nutritious and life-extending, all of which might well find a welcome on any gourmet's diet.

And now for the HOW of the defender fats—the ways in which they guard your health. The polyunsaturated fats play an important role in actually strengthening your capillary walls. When atherosclerosis develops, new tiny blood vessels form within the cholesterol deposits in the arteries. These tiny capillaries may rupture—burst—and the clot formed in this way will further narrow an already partially obstructed, and perhaps vital, blood vessel.

If this happens in a coronary artery, partial closure may be completed, cutting off the blood supply to part of the heart muscle. This is called a coronary heart attack, and it may be abruptly or gradually fatal. Sudden death is a chilling picture. Look upon it now—and every time you see a hot fudge sundae, a piece of candy, a slice of bread, any sugar or starch food, see "sudden death" descending on you! This awareness of danger may save *your* life.

Since the polyunsaturated oils strengthen your capillary walls and decrease their fragility, they give you protection against sudden rupture of these tiny vessels. Since you have only recently learned the facts about the Longevity Diet, and have only now begun to put your new knowledge into action, you probably have cholesterol deposits in your arteries right now (but not for long if you are faithful to your goal of 100 years!). Since this is so, the Cantor Cocktail is your lifeline into the future. It contains, among other essential nutrients, the defender fats that will help you rid yourself of those cholesterol deposits while strengthening your capillary walls, especially the capillaries in your present cholesterol deposits.

The Mysterious Ways of the Defender Fats

The exact mechanism by which the defender fats lower your blood cholesterol is not known. There are many studies now in progress, and we will probably have answers soon. For us the important point is that the polyunsaturated fats do indeed "remove" cholesterol from the arteries. The unsaturated vegetable and fish oils do lower blood cholesterol levels. They do reverse atherosclerosis. They do improve capillary strength. That is all we need to know in order to move confidently toward our goal of 100 years and greater vitality each day of those years.

Substitution of Defender Fats is Your Success Key

Aside from cutting calories by the half-portion method, and the virtual elimination of sugars and starches, *the most important part of the Longevity Diet is for you to always substitute the "defender" fats for the "killer" fats.* This means that the most important foods for you from now on will be safflower oil, corn oil, and seafood.

The average American diet is 40 to 60 per cent fat (in terms of total calories), including both saturated and unsaturated fats. You must try to reduce this to 20 to 25 per cent, and the Longevity Diet will show you how to accomplish this.

You won't need to count calories, if you don't want to, although calories do count, as you now know. I am not a calorie counter, and I don't expect you to be one either. Nor do I expect you to weigh and measure all foods. All I ask you to do is to learn the principles of the Longevity Diet, think about them until they become second nature to you, use them every day until they replace your previous patterns of eating death-dealing foods, and you will never need to count calories or to weigh foods. You will automatically eat the right foods in the right amounts, and you will do it with satisfaction and pleasure. Your pleasure will mount every time you look into a mirror, and every time you hear the compliments of your friends.

Don't Bring Home the Bacon

The typical American breakfast of bacon and eggs, buttered toast and creamed coffee is the first "habit" you must abandon— once and for all. This is the Killer Breakfast, since it is very high both in cholesterol and calories. You can help yourself to health right now by substituting a Defender Breakfast for the Killer Breakfast. There are many ways to do this, all of them pleasant and filling. Take your choice.

For example, you may have your eggs simply by eliminating the yolks. My personal preference is for the whites of two hard boiled eggs. I grant you that it was difficult for me to make the change at the very outset, since I had been eating two soft boiled eggs for breakfast for over 30 years. But I was faced with the choice of life or death, and I decided not to commit suicide. So I stopped firing the slow cholesterol bullets by *learning to like* the whites of hard boiled eggs, in that way providing a good grade protein for breakfast and retaining the emotional pattern of "eggs" for breakfast. You can do the same. At no point will I ask you to do what I have not already done, and what I have already proved to be effective in my own medical experience.

Do you insist upon bread? Okay, then take a slice of a good whole wheat or other dark (but not artificially darkened) or whole grain bread. If you are overweight and find your emotional patterns demanding bread, stay with the profile-type bread, the high protein type designed just for the fatties who refuse to face the facts of life with unsheathed willpower. Want butter on your bread? Okay, use one of the safflower or corn oil margarines, choosing one that is high in the polyunsaturated fats and only partially hydrogenated (see page 173). Spread it on your slice of breakfast bread. Satisfied? Do you want coffee? Alright, but take it dark or with skimmed milk. It tastes the same when you substitute skimmed milk for the deadly cream. Realizing that this will save your life, it should taste better! Use one of the sugar substitutes instead of the denatured, empty calories of ordinary white sugar. Or learn to drink your coffee without sugar.

Try one of the *decaffeinated coffees* if you want to protect your heart and nervous system against an overdose of caffeine. If you were blindfolded, or if this coffee were served to you without telling you that it wasn't regular coffee, you probably wouldn't know the difference. I will tell you more about the dangers of coffee in a later consultation. Or use a substitute beverage like one brewed from certain roasted cereal grains. It can be Postum—a good, tasty, healthful drink. I like it. Or how about buttermilk? Do you want orange juice or half a grapefruit? Okay, no holds barred, but don't forget that these fruits contain sugar. Since it is a natural sugar, it is less harmful than the ordinary white sugar (but keep the calories in mind, especially if you are carrying extra pounds of fat around with you).

Are you a cereal eater? Alright, but take a whole grain cereal (perhaps steel cut oatmeal) with skimmed milk. Again, you must watch your total calories if you are overweight. A simple rule for those of you who are overweight is to let the scales tell you if you are "doing something right." If you are losing one to three pounds a week, "you must be doing something right," to paraphrase a popular television advertisement. If you are not losing those extra pounds consistently, cut down on the size of your portions—and watch those sugars and starches. Well, how's that for a breakfast menu? Do you still feel deprived? I don't think so, for the Longevity Diet, when properly applied, is a very adequate, very satisfying diet. It satisfies me, in spite of my gourmet tastes.

The Golden Rule of Moderation

Moderation will always be your keynote. It will always be the keystone of the arch of long life and good health. Although I certainly do not advise it, you can even take small doses of arsenic in moderation, and gradually build up a tolerance to this deadly poison. The Borgias of historic fame used to do this so they could serve wine with a heavy dose of arsenic in it to their enemies, while drinking it themselves to throw their "guests" off guard. What I am trying to say is that you can even take the deadly foods in moderation, although I am not recommending this except during your "slips," and I hope they will not come too often.

I go further, and say that moderation should guide you even when you are eating the defender foods. For example, I want you to limit the total amount of fat in your diet. I want you to do this even if your entire fat intake is polyunsaturated. Too much of a good thing is often just as bad as too much of a bad thing. That is where the half-portion idea comes in. And as your stomach returns to normal size, you will require less and less food to satisfy your appetite.

And so we come to calories, and I want to say a little more about that before leaving the subject for all time.

What Is a Calorie?

First, let me repeat that *calories do count*. They count so much that they can kill you if you take too many of them. We overcome this, not by counting calories, but by moderation in eating, and by eliminating the high calorie sugars and starches, while limiting the total of the even higher calorie fats.

The calorie used in the study of life functions (metabolism) is the large calorie. This is simply the amount of heat required to raise one kilogram of water from 15 to 16 degrees centigrade. *Calorie* is simply a word which designates the energy required for all of your body processes. Instead of using an electrical term for measurement, although our bodies give off electricity constantly, we use a heat term to measure the amount of heat given off during all body functions. That is all a calorie is—a unit of heat measurement. You won't find it in any food as a part of the food substance, for it is neither a protein, a carbohydrate nor a fat; neither is it a vitamin or a mineral. It is simply a way to tell how much energy a particular food supplies and how much energy our body requires.

The large calorie, as above defined, is actually a kilo-calorie— 1,000 small calories. But it is the one we must consider when we talk about our own metabolism. Small or large, it is simply a measure for energy.

The caloric values given for all foods are only averages, since there is great variation. For example, animal proteins appear to yield higher values than the plant proteins. Animal fats give more calories than dairy fats. But the average caloric value, the average amount of energy you will get from the three main classes of foods is as follows:

Protein	4.1 calories per gram
Carbohydrate	4.1 calories per gram
Fats	9.3 calories per gram

How Many Calories Do You Need?

Now we come to the life and death question, the question of how many calories you actually need. Again, I can only give you averages based upon age, sex, and so forth. And also upon the type of work you do. And I must caution you that the calorie contents of food differ with so many factors that we will again only be dealing with rough and changing averages.

The number of calories (energy) you and I require is obviously based upon the amount of energy needed to keep our normal body functions going and the amount of energy over and above that we need for our daily activities. The amount we need for our normal body functions naturally depends upon how big we are, how old we are and our sex. The amount of energy we need for our work depends on the nature of the work—how hard we work. Simple enough? The Committee on Caloric Requirements of the Food and Agriculture Organization of the United Nations offers the following *average* figures.

ESTIMATE OF CALORIC REQUIREMENTS OF ADULTS ACCORDING TO SIZE

Weight	Men	Women	Pregnant Women	Lactating Women
88	. . . .	1823	2273	2823
99	2447	1987	2437	2987
110	2643	2146	2596	3146
121	2833	2300	2750	3300
132	3019	2451	2901	3451
143	3200	2599	3049	3599
154	3379	2743	3193	3743
165	3553			
176	3725			

These are the required calories per day when the average temperature is 50 degrees Fahrenheit. You see, the outside temperature is also a factor in determining how many calories you need. Obviously, your body needs more energy when it is very cold in order to keep warm.

And now let us take a look at how many calories you need at various ages.

REQUIRED CALORIES ACCORDING TO AGE—ADULTS

Age	Men	Women
20-30	3200	2300
30-40	3104	2231
40-50	3008	2162
50-60	2765	1990
60-70	2528	1817
70	2208	1587

If you are over 70, don't worry about calories. Just follow the half-portion rule, and the other rules of the Longevity Diet, and you have a very good chance of reaching and surpassing the century mark.

Learn the Calorie Lessons Now

Notice that you need less and less calories as you move along through the years. Notice also that I do not say, "As you grow older," since I do not intend that you will grow older as time passes. Rather, it is my desire that you grow younger, both internally and externally.

Most of us tend to eat more as we become able to afford more. But the really wise are the ones who eat less, regardless of how much they can afford to eat. Watch the patrons of a fashionable restaurant, for they are usually well informed and want to stay alive long enough to spend and enjoy their wealth. They will usually forego the appetizer, begin their meal with a salad, and then have a single, simply cooked dish—usually fowl or fish. There is usually no dessert for them. They can afford it from the cost point of view, but they can't afford it from the staying-alive point of view.

I have just described dinner—a very good and healthful dinner. You could enjoy that, couldn't you, and feel well satisfied, content and pleased with the knowledge that you have enjoyed a healthful meal?

Calories Needed for Various Types of Work

And now we shall take a quick look at the number of calories you need for different types of activities (average estimates only).

ACTIVITY	CALORIES USED UP PER HOUR
Dressing or Undressing	33
Sitting and Doing Nothing	16
Standing and Doing Nothing	20
Walking	150 to 200
Running	500 to 950
Dishwashing	60
Sewing	60
Ironing	60
Sweeping	110
Knitting	30
Mental Activity	6 to 8
Writing	10 to 20
Home Hobby Carpentry	100 to 200
Sawing Wood	400
A Good Typist	15 to 45
Painting a Room	150
Bicycling	150 to 300
Swimming	200 to 750
Wrestling	1000

To give you an idea of how rough these figures are, another reliable source offers the following:

ACTIVITY	CALORIES PER HOUR
Sewing	110
Typing	140
Housework	150
Carpentry	240

The Work-Calorie Lesson for Your Guidance

What I want you to realize is that you probably don't need anywhere near the amount of calories you are now eating. When you eat half portions, you are probably coming nearer to your actual needs. Certainly you are getting further from the danger zone of excess calories, excess pounds, and excess strain on your heart.

How Many Calories Do YOU Need?

See how difficult it is to set a definite figure? There are too many variables—outside temperature (room or outdoors), your body weight and skin surface area, your age, your sex, your general condition, your moment-to-moment activity, and so forth. It even varies with age, with the degree of emotional stress, and with an infinity of varying factors throughout the course of a single day.

Let us simply say that if you are overweight you are obviously taking too many calories. In simple words, you are eating too much, and probably the wrong foods as well. If you are losing weight, and don't want to, you are probably not eating enough (or you have an overactive thyroid gland, or some other body disturbance). Your emotions can make you overeat or undereat, whether you are sick or well.

Check your weight against the ideal standards (see page 144), and then act accordingly. You will probably find that the half-portion idea is for you. And you will undoubtedly find that you will move toward the ideal level as soon as you start on the Longevity Diet. In other words—*watch pounds, not calories!* And that's enough about calories—at least for this consultation.

More Tips on Enjoying Life In Living Longer

And now for a few more tips on how to enjoy and make your life more productive and creative in living a longer life. Since your emotions cause most of the diseases men are heir to, learn more about yourself. Read books on psychosomatic disturbances and learn the way your body talks to you in terms of symptoms. This is called *organ language,* and if you want to know more about the way your emotions prevent you from truly enjoying life, I would suggest that you drop me a note at the UNITROL Teaching Institute.* I will send you a list of the books you should read, books that will show

---

*The UNITROL Teaching Institute, 147-41 Sanford Ave., Flushing, N.Y. 11355.

you how to rid yourself of your emotionally-based, psychosomatic
health wreckers. Once you have done this, you will be well on your
way to happier and healthier living. Until then, take my word for
the fact that most illness is emotionally induced. Since a fault
known is already half cured, once you recognize that fact that most
of your complaints are probably psychosomatic you will have taken
the first giant step toward correction of those problems. And once
you rid yourself of your emotional problems, you will be ready for
happier as well as healthier living.

Right now, turn to pages 179-189 in the Second Key for more information on how your emotions cause symptoms and body changes,
even serious disease, and how to control them.

Learn to replace your IPB's with MPB's—your Immature Patterns of Behavior with Mature Patterns of Behavior. For example,
the child takes and never gives. Adults, and especially parents, love
to give things to their children. But you are no longer a child. Learn
to replace this IPB with the MPB of giving. Give of yourself, your
time, your understanding, and your wisdom to those who need and
will benefit from those fine qualities. You will have fun doing it, I
promise you. You will feel fulfilled. Life will be better, happier,
more soul-satisfying. When you help others, you help yourself even
more.

Replace the IPB of anger and hatred, bigotry and intolerance,
with the MPB's of kindness, good will toward all men, gentleness
and understanding. Learn to turn the other cheek, and you will be
preventing the high blood pressure, the stroke, the coronary closure
of stress. You see, as I have told you, your IPB's are causing emotionally-based, stress symptoms and body changes—changes we call
psychosomatic disease. And when you substitute MPB's for your
childish IPB's, you rid yourself of the symptoms, allow your body to
heal itself, and you become a better, a happier and a healthier person. You do this while being of service to your fellowman and to
your community.

Bend and You Won't Break

Learn to be more flexible, and to change with the rapidly changing times. After all, we are living in the space age, and if you wish
to be truly young—both in body and mind—you must adapt and

change, become part of the space age. Give up the IPB of rigidity and substitute the MPB of flexibility. Bend so you will not break, and bend with the times, move with the current, stay in the main-stream of life.

Think Young

I am telling you to become part of the youth of your area, join in their activities, and learn to *think young* and *act young*. You are as young as you think. Always remember that.

And NOW, in summary . . .

1. You have learned more about the defender fats, and how they protect you against the deadly killer fats.
2. You know that simple diet changes can lower your blood cholesterol level and rid your arteries of their dangerous partial blockage by cholesterol deposits.
3. I have taught you the simple rules to rid yourself of excess and dangerous pounds, the use of the natural appetite-depressant, and why more normal weight is essential to long life and better health.
4. You now know about the very simple blood tests for cholesterol level and for the protein-bound iodine estimation of thyroid function.
5. You know why you must avoid rapid weight gain once you have lost those unsightly pounds, and why this up and down weight fluctuation is dangerous for your heart and arteries.
6. I have introduced you to other patients who point up these dangers for you so you can avoid them in your own Longevity Program.
7. I have introduced you to the "moderate slip" concept to make your diet easier and your life more pleasant.
8. You now know about the subconscious and the conscious resistances, and how to overcome them.
9. I have told you to "be human and be happy," and have showed you how to do that.
10. You have learned about the Killer Breakfast, and how to

substitute the delicious and very filling Defender Breakfast.

11. You have learned the golden rule of moderation.

12. Once and for all, you know the facts about calories, and
    that calories do count, although I don't want you to count
    them.

13. You know that it is better to watch pounds than to watch
    calories. This is so much simpler and so much better for
    you that it is a wonder that no one ever thought of it be-
    fore. The secret is now yours to guide you into longer life,
    healthier life, and happier living.

14. I have given you more tips on how to enjoy life, and I
    have shown you how to substitute the important and con-
    structive MPB's for the destructive and health-retarding
    IPB's.

CHAPTER 7

HOW TO AVOID
THE DEADLY WORK
OF KILLER FATS

I do hope that you are following all the advice I have given you to this point. If you are not, you are cheating only yourself. I enjoy talking to you, and you are paying a fee for these services, but they are not going to do you the maximum good unless you put everything you are learning into prompt action.

I hope that you have started on the half-portion method for the reduction of your calories. If you have, you probably have noticed that it is taking less and less food to satisfy your appetite. That is because your stomach is going back to its normal, smaller size— the size that it was before you began distending it with enormous portions and many-course meals.

You probably also have begun to enjoy the weight loss that is restoring your previous youthful figure and face. Wonderful! You have also begun to cut down on starches and to eliminate all sugars. That is the quickest and the best route to a low caloric diet and a new youthful face and figure.

At the same time I am sure that you are now taking your Cantor Cocktail before each meal, both for its appetite-satisfying action and for its polyunsaturated oil content. You have certainly cut down on animal and dairy fats, and have substituted the vegetable oils, especially the safflower oil products.

Are you drinking at least six to eight glasses of water each day? Most patients have trouble with this very simple rule, so don't feel too bad if you are a little slow in developing this important habit. Take a mineral-vitamin tablet or capsule meanwhile, especially if you must drink soft water instead of the natural, mineralized hard water.

And finally, are you enjoying life? Change your thinking over to the positive side, and learn to have fun each day. Never refuse the opportunity to have a good time. Spend more time with the young at heart, and less with the old fogey rocking-chair set. There is plenty of time for that when you are over 120.

What Are the Killer Fats?

And now I want to tell you more about the killer fats. Of course you already know that *these are the hard fats, the fully hydrogenated fats, the animal and dairy product fats*. You will find them in all meats and in butter, whole milk, cream, the hard cheeses and other dairy products.

By this time you are so well informed about their dangers that the very mention of hard fats—meat and dairy foods—starts you thinking of coronary heart attacks and strokes. That's good. We want the very sight of such foods to trigger this automatic reaction. The more emotional you get about such foods, the more you *fear* their obvious danger, their threat to your very existence, the easier it will be for you to say, "No, thank you," every time they are offered to you. Always remember that when there is a battle between your emotions and your intellect, it will be the emotions that will win. So gear your fear emotions to set you against the hard fat, killer fat foods. This will give you the best possible eating habits, since your emotions and your intellect will be truly in gear, both telling you that you must stay away from the killer fats if you are to avoid having a suicide case history as the last chapter in your life.

Searching for the Killer Fats

The search for the killer fats is a detective story worth recounting. It is the detective work that medicine calls epidemiology. This is a fancy word to cover the detective work that traces patterns of disease throughout the entire world—a kind of international detective agency staffed entirely by physicians and their allies. The detective work I will now tell you about proves that patterns of diet and disease can be traced throughout the entire world, and that these patterns clearly indict the hard fats as killer fats.

The men of the epidemiology detective staff study whole populations and the patterns of disease in those populations. Just as the safe-cracker follows a set pattern of operation that makes it possible for the Safe and Loft Squad of a large city police force to identify a "job" by the way it was carried out, so disease leaves its characteristic pattern wherever it strikes. As a matter of fact—and this is of vital importance to you—the major clues for the cause of the number one killer diseases, the heart and blood vessel "epidemic," came from population pattern studies.

What type of questions do these medical detectives ask? The epidemiologist wants to know whether the number of coronary cases varies from country to country. Do the number of cases vary from time to time? Do we have more coronary disease now, for example, than we had 25 or 50 years ago? Was there more or less during times of general undernutrition—times when whole populations had less than enough food to eat? Do more of the younger and middle-aged group die of coronary disease in some countries than in others? And here is an important question—one that might not occur to you—is it better to be rich or poor? In terms of heart disease, is there a difference between the desk worker and the ditch digger? (With today's wage scale in the United States, I'm not certain which of these is "rich.") And what about the difference between men and women? Which sex suffers most from atherosclerosis? Is there a difference between the white man and the Negro? Many, many questions must be asked by the medical detectives, and the answers must be obtained from whole populations, not just from a small sample. Quite a job, but they did it! And that is not all.

What Are the Clues in This Search for Health?

The territory that must be checked for clues includes not only the entire population area, but also the climate, income, diet, occupation, and race. This is quite a jigsaw puzzle. The medical detectives did quite a job, and came up with all the answers. You have already learned some of the answers, and you will learn still more as we see each other during these consultations. I will tell you now, even before we begin our detective story, that the relationship between cholesterol-fat metabolism and hardening of the arteries by atherosclerosis is so well documented by the epidemiologist as to be beyond question. And now for our brief panoramic survey of the world-wide jigsaw puzzle. We will take another moment, before starting, to tell you about a family problem that will interest you and will show you, in capsule form, how the total picture must be considered.

A Family Case History That Might Relate to Your Family

This family of "suicide-seekers" with a "license to kill" themselves by overeating (a license we all have!) consisted of a horribly overweight mother, a very slender father, and one son and one daughter. An ideal family, except for their eating habits and their physical condition.

Let's start with the mother. She was 50 years old chronologically, and 90 years old in body. She had severe atherosclerosis, with pain in the chest whenever she attempted "more than a little housework." She had a blood pressure in the stratosphere and damaged kidney function to match that. She was a hefty 210 pounds despite her five-foot-one height. Not a pretty picture, but very common in these high starch, high fat diet days. That was the diet this family favored, and they could not be easily budged from it because it was the way "mother used to cook." Once again, the battle between the emotions and the intellect was lost to the emotions.

Dad was a salaried worker who had a physically active job. This was his life-line, since—as you will learn later—exercise helps cut down the blood cholesterol level. He ate well, the same diet as the rest of the family, but only when at home—and his job kept him away from home for lunch. He had a moderately overactive thyroid gland, and this helped him burn up the empty calories of the high starch and high sugar diet he had at family meals.

Daughter was a younger replica of her mother. Her blood pressure was on its way up at 20 years of age, and her diet had lost no time in making her 60 pounds overweight. Son took after mother also, unfortunately. His blood pressure was normal but his blood cholesterol level was in orbit!

The Lessons of This Case History

Here we have a miniature population study—a family population. We see the effect of a family pattern of eating. Mother and dad—but especially mother—set the pattern for each of us (except for the family rebels who refuse to do anything mother orders). We see the effect of a high fat, high starch, high sugar diet with far too many calories. We see the effect of age and sex, and the pattern of disease resulting from the eating patterns.

This family had another diet pattern that was potentially dangerous and part of the typical food suicide pattern—*the overflowing coffee pot*. Two, three, and four cups with each meal was the usual. Later on you will see that when you go over five cups per day you are asking for serious trouble. More than five cups of coffee a day increases the chance of a heart attack!

You now have enough information on this food suicide family to know that they were already exercising their "license to kill" by aiming many slow bullets at their own vital organs. Mother was directing the firing squad.

Learn the lessons of this family, and give up your own license to kill yourself. Learn the lessons of this miniature epidemiologic study and stop firing the cholesterol-calorie-coffee bullets at your own vital organs.

Just a few concluding words, and we will leave this family. Finally, after many ups and downs, they followed the Longevity Diet patterns, and are now on their way to better health and longer life. They certainly look much better, especially the ladies of the family. Released from their fortress of fat, they are now quite attractive, and daughter is much happier since her new figure and face are attracting the boys in ever-increasing numbers.

What Happened When "They Lived Off The Fat of The Land"?

It is interesting to note that the Old Testament was right when it reported that, "They lived off the fat of the land." (*Genesis 45,*

17-18.) We see evidence of this when we study the mummies of Egyptian nobility and their priesthood, and find that there was advanced atherosclerosis in their main-line heart arteries. *The rich lived well, but they didn't live long,* even in those days. The rich know better today, but fortunately you don't have to be rich to eat the Longevity Diet, especially since the cheaper cuts of meat are the safest, and since fish is not too expensive in most parts of the world.

What about the average man? The staples of Egyptian times, even as now, were bread, potatoes and rice. The noted medical historian, H. E. Sigerist, tells us that in the Egypt of the Pharaohs the staples of the common people were bread and beer. Naturally we don't have preserved mummies of the common people of those days, but it is a safe bet that this type of *undernutrition* probably prevented atherosclerosis. We can make that bet based on the statistics we have from the economically underdeveloped countries of Asia, Africa, and Latin America.

How Are Things In Good Old U.S.A.?

What about the United States? With all our wealth, all our subsidies for farmers, our enormous food supply, our caves full of overflow butter, our granaries full of overstocked wheat, our advanced knowledge—certainly we must be better off in our health patterns. Don't you believe it. If anything, we are in greater danger as a result of the very abundance that surrounds us. The death rate from heart and artery disease in the United States is appalling. We lose the flower of our youth and the best of our executive level men and women, as well as the experience and creativity of the middle-age men and women, in truly epidemic proportions every year. War casualties are very small compared to heart and artery disease casualties. And it is all due to the killer fats in the rich American diet, added to the empty calorie content.

Killer Fats of the U.S.A.

In the United States we have an abundance of these killer fats in the marbled steaks and other meats, butter, eggs and cheese. When we add to this the empty calories of candy, refined white sugar, and white bread, we can understand the reason for the epidemic proportions of coronary heart disease in our country (1,000 cases per 100,000 males age 45 to 64). Let that sink in, and see if you still want these killer fat foods. Ponder that, and see if you still think the empty calories are worth the price. No one in his right mind wants to become an early death statistic, and you must decide, once and for all, if you are indeed in your right mind, or if you are destined to become a food suicide statistic.

Diet and Length of Life

There is a clearly defined relationship between the food you eat and the number of years you will live. Our epidemiology detectives showed us this in 1924. Based on observations made in China, Egypt, India, East Africa and Malaya, as compared with comparable studies in other parts of the world, including the United States, Austria and Germany, the conclusion was drawn that, "In no race for which a high cholesterol intake (in the form of eggs, butter and milk) and fat intake are recorded is atherosclerosis absent." Let me translate that gobbledygook for you. In simple words, a high cholesterol and fat diet always causes atherosclerosis—heart and artery disease—in every country studied.

But, "Where a high protein diet is consumed, which naturally contains small quantities of cholesterol, but where the neutral fat intake is low, atherosclerosis is not prevalent." Again, translation, please. Simply stated, those who eat a high protein diet, little fat, and little or no cholesterol, do not develop artherosclerosis.

Since atherosclerosis in heart arteries and other arteries is the basis for the number one killer in our society, you certainly won't reach your 100-year goal by eating the killer fats! Just think a moment. If these observations, published in the prestigious and well circulated AMA *Archives of Pathology,* had been acted upon by physicians and their patients, millions of deaths from atherosclerotic heart disease might have been prevented or postponed for many years. Remember that these conclusions were published in 1924!

To Be Rich Is to Have Better Health?

This very same study by the same medical detective (S. R. Rosenthal) showed that in India and Egypt atherosclerosis was rare among the very poor. Their diet was largely cereal. But the number one killer took deadly aim with his cholesterol bullets among those who could afford a diet high in the killer fats and cholesterol. It is this type of detective work that pinpoints diet rather than race or climate as the cause of the epidemic proportions of heart and artery disease.

It's the Food You Eat Regardless of the Country Where You Were Born

Sheng was a very young Chinese boy, 18 years old when I first saw him. He had just come to this country, and was working in a Chinese restaurant. His boss, who had required rectal surgery some years before, sent the youngster to me since he had a painful rectal condition. I corrected the problem in the usual way, in my office, removing an anal ulcer and sending him back to work the next day. His general health was excellent at that time, nevertheless.

I saw him again ten years later. This time he had a very high blood cholesterol, diabetes and high blood pressure, as well as the overactive bowel of stress. His psychosomatic organ language was speaking with a loud and clear voice.

Now it is quite usual for the average Chinese to have low blood cholesterol and a low incidence of heart and artery disease. But that is when they are on the simple rice diet of their native land, with plenty of fish, and only occasional meat. Sheng had adapted to his new country by adopting the American diet as well as the American way of life. His killer fat intake was the same as that of the average American, and it was doing its deadly job, regardless of his health inheritance from his native land.

After I showed him how he was inadvertently committing suicide, he changed his eating habits promptly, and became both healthier and younger once again. This illustrates that it is the food that counts, and not where you were born. Death takes no holiday and plays no favorites.

Watch that Blood Cholesterol if You Are Financially Well Off

Blood cholesterol level studies can be closely related to the number of heart and artery fatalities in all countries. The people of the less developed countries again get the better of the deal. In the United States, and in all countries where a high fat and high caloric diet can be afforded, the blood cholesterol level rises higher and higher with each decade of adult life. In the underdeveloped countries where the people cannot afford meat and dairy products, they have a relatively low blood cholesterol level and very little atherosclerotic heart and artery disease.

The medical detectives have traced this fatal connection between blood cholesterol level and heart and artery disease all over the world. They learned that this ever-increasing level of blood cholesterol is not found in the South African Bantu, but is very prevalent in the more privileged South African Europeans whose diet is rich in calories, total fats and cholesterol.

A famous comedian used to wow his audiences by saying, "I've been rich and I've been poor, and believe me—rich is better." (*I wonder!*)

We don't find a high blood cholesterol level or much heart and artery disease in manual laborers in Guatamala and India, for they are largely vegetarians. But we do find both in the "better off" physicians, businessmen, officials and army officers who indulge in a high calorie, high total fat, high saturated fat diet.

And so our far-ranging fact-collecting medical detectives bring us the evidence from the far corners of the earth. And with the evidence, they bring the opportunity for better health and longer life for all who listen and take heed. Once again—take heed and take heart (and forgive another very serious pun).

What Is "Normal?"

I have already pointed out that I do not consider the American laboratory standards of "normal" to be valid. I do not believe that it is normal to have a blood cholesterol level of up to 250 mg. per 100 cc. of blood when such a level is associated with an epidemic level of heart and artery disease.

All the evidence of our best epidemiologists—our best medical detectives—agrees with me. The *best* serum cholesterol level is obviously much lower than the levels considered statistically normal in the United States. I would like to see *your* level at 150 mg. per 100 cc. of blood. I would like to see you keep it there, since this is the level associated with the lowest level of heart and artery disease.

It is now quite obvious to you that if you are to prolong your life into the 100-year or more range—for that matter, if you are to stay alive at all—you must avoid becoming a heart and artery statistic. Get out of the self-killing by wrong eating class right now, and stay out of it by staying on the Longevity Diet pattern.

The Medical Detective and the Best Diet

What foods are eaten by those whose blood cholesterol level is low and who have very little or no heart and artery disease? This is the final question we must ask our disease detectives. We have already mentioned cereals and potatoes, and we have learned that *the cereal and potato eaters have little or no killer fat in their diet.*

In Scandinavia and the Low Countries during World War II (during the time of the German Occupation), there was a marked decline in atherosclerotic heart disease. This was associated with an equally marked decrease in calories, total fats, saturated fats and cholesterol! Obviously there wasn't much to eat during that difficult time, and certainly little of the high solid fat meat and dairy products.

But by 1950 the picture had changed. The dietary restrictions were a thing of the past, and once again both meat and dairy products became more plentiful. So did high blood cholesterol levels and heart and artery disease! Convinced? You should be.

It's Important to Remember:

Our diet and death detectives lead us to very important conclusions.

They teach us that the *vegetarian diet is best,* with certain modifications to suit the needs of our society and the principles of the Longevity Diet—your first Key to Longevity. Although you may eat meat in small portions, the less the better. Choose lean cuts of beef, cut off all obvious fat, and burn out the rest by cooking it to "well done."

Better still, *choose fowl and veal rather than beef.* Remember that white meat has less fat than dark meat. Chicken and turkey are safer than the fatty duck.

Avoid whole milk and cream. Skimmed milk and buttermilk are okay. Stay away from the processed cheeses no matter what the television commercials tell you.

Eat no butter. Substitute the equally tasty soft margarines. Enjoy fruits, vegetables and most nuts. Eat two large, mixed green vegetable salads every day, using safflower oil and lemon juice (with garlic if you like) for your salad dressing.

Eat fish every day—especially the ocean fish. Here you have the very best defender fats. Enjoy crabmeat, lobster and all other sea food, if you like. Dip your lobster meat in melted soft margarine. How's that for your gourmet diet?

Start your meal with a shrimp or lobster or crabmeat cocktail with cocktail sauce, if you are really that hungry. (I doubt that you will be after your appetite-depressant Cantor Cocktail!) Follow with fish, fowl or lean meat (veal is especially safe), and a large mixed green vegetable salad.

I would suggest that you fill your stomach and cut your appetite still further by having the salad before your main course. If you must have dessert, make it angel food cake, a water sherbet, or fruit.

Do you drool over fried foods? Okay, fry your fish or chicken in the magical safflower oil.

I will have more details about the Longevity Diet in another chapter, during another consultation, but I thought you ought to have some mouth-watering conclusions after this death-detective story. It's all very interesting, but you need to know what to do about all this evidence. And what you can do about it is to enjoy three gourmet meals every day, having fun all the way through the next 100 years, BUT ALWAYS REMEMBER THE GOLDEN RULE OF MODERATION!

More Tips on Having Fun and Living Creatively

- Learn to think *fun*. *Think* fun and you will have fun.
- Learn to think *young*. *Think* young and you will be young.
- Learn to think *good health*. *Think* good health and your subconscious mind will put the necessary glands and other body tissues to work to make you healthy.
- Learn to think *success*. *Think* success and plan accordingly.

Then put your plans into action. Plans without action to match are not worth much.

- Think *action*, and stop sitting around waiting for the fruits of success to fall into your lap. You have to get up, stand on your own two feet, and *shake the tree.*
- Always remember that the helping hand you are looking for is at the end of your own arm. Action and still more action, if you want to be a success, have fun, and shed those unwanted years.
- Stop sitting around and vegetating. That's the road to early senility and an early grave.
- Get interested in everything, learn something new every day, and *do something new* every day.

And NOW, in summary . . .

1. You have learned the world-wide facts about the killer fats.
2. You know the evidence that incriminates the killer fats in the world-wide epidemic of heart and artery deaths.
3. You have seen the meat and dairy fats—the universal killer fats—at their deadly work in every country of the world. You have traveled the world over with the medical detectives, the epidemiologists, to track down the killer fats.
4. I have also introduced you to the coffee-pot cause of sudden death.
5. Your world-ranging studies with the medical detectives have shown you the life-saving importance of cutting calories and eliminating sugars, starch and the killer fats.
6. You have learned that the vegetarian diet is best for those countries where they cannot afford other foods. But I have given you a modified vegetarian diet that is best for you and full of fun-foods.
7. In the U.S.A., you now know, the only way to reach your goal of 100 or more years is to stop "living off the fat of the land."
8. Your world-wide adventures have proved that diet is the determining factor in length of life.

9. You now know the truth about the so-called normal level of blood cholesterol, and the fact that it is not "normal" at all.

10. I have shown you more of the gourmet quality of the Longevity Diet, and have given you foods to drool over— all good for your health.

11. And finally, I have given you more tips on having fun and living creatively.

CHAPTER 8

WHAT TO DO ABOUT AVOIDING THE ATHEROSCLEROSIS THREAT

Once again we return to my consulting room, this time to tell you more about the five main components of the atherosclerosis puzzle, and the many little pieces of the jigsaw of threatening death. First, however, since I want to be sure that you are fully up-to-date on our consultations to this point, let's review what I expect from you.

To This Point

If you have been following my advice to this point, you are feeling better than you have in many years. You are becoming slimmer (if you were overweight), your skin looks healthier and your complexion is better. You have greater vitality, and you are beginning to become more aware of really *living*. You are now eating half-portions or less. You do not have any desire for more, since your stomach is now back to normal size. Besides, your Cantor Cocktail before each meal is acting as the best kind of normal appetite depressant. At the same time, it is giving you the polyunsaturated fat you need to rid your arteries of their deadly cholesterol deposits.

You are *enjoying* ocean fish each day. You no longer can stand the sight of the deadly meat and dairy product fat—the ugly fat that sends its unerring cholesterol bullets into your vital heart and arteries.

You are drinking six to eight glasses of water each day—hard water if possible. Or you are supplementing your water quota with a vitamin-mineral capsule or tablet.

You are free from bondage to the immature pattern of sugar—the candy, cake, and ice cream rewards of your childhood. And you now eat very little starch, in order to cut down on total calories. Very good!

And, perhaps best of all, I am glad to know that you are beginning to enjoy life, to think and act young.

Let's go on now to tell you more about the First Key to Longevity, the nutrition key, and at the same time we will add the other major interrelated causes of artery and heart disease.

The Chart of Sudden Death

To make it easy for you, I have prepared a chart to show the various factors that fire the slow bullets into the vital organs. You will, of course, be able to refer to this chart whenever you wish. It will help you to avoid becoming a food suicide statistic. It will guide you on the path to reaching an age of 100 or more years.

SUDDEN DEATH CHART
(Slow Suicide For Many)

1. *Dietary Imbalance*

    Overnutrition:

    > empty calories in excess
    > excess total calories
    > excess total fats
    > excess saturated fats
    > excess cholesterol
    > excess refined carbohydrates
    > excess salt

    Undernutrition:

    > insufficient bulk
    > insufficient vitamins and minerals

insufficient unsaturated fats
(essential fatty acids)
insufficient amino acids

Deficiency may be relative or absolute

2. *Obesity*

3. *Hypertension*

4. *Tobacco (cigarette smoking)*

5. *Stress*

Stages of Damage:

Dietary Imbalance → Hypercholesterolemia
Hypercholesterolemia + Obesity + Hypertension → Arteriosclerotic Heart
Disease
(This is the chain of events which occurs especially in middle age males.)
Dietary Imbalance alone, without obesity or hypertension → High Incidence of Coronary Artery Disease.

Interpretation of the Above Chart

And now let's translate this into everyday language, and tell you exactly what you must do to avoid these slow and sudden bullets of food suicide. I will illustrate with a case history from my files, so you can see how some of these factors actually work to kill the unaware, or the uncooperative.

A housewife of 37 had let herself get fat immediately after marriage. She had a strong family history of diabetes, her father having died from this disease when he was in his early forties. There was no evidence of diabetes when I saw her; her blood sugar was quite normal and there was no sugar spilling into her urine.

She did have a very high cholesterol level, consistently over 350 mg. per 100 cc. of blood, and I advised her of the importance of a proper diet. She already knew that she was probably predisposed to develop diabetes, and I emphasized the life-or-death necessity to lose the extra pounds to guard herself against the dangers of heart and artery disaster. She appeared to understand, but chose to exercise her "license to kill," with herself as the target.

The slow bullets gathered speed as she continued on her hard fat, high caloric route, and she died of a stroke three years later. Suicide? Yes!

Chart Your Own Life Line

You needn't study the life-line on your palm to know how long you will live. You need only refer to the SUDDEN DEATH (Slow Suicide) chart, pick out the factors that apply to you, decide whether or not you will eliminate them by following my instructions, and you will be able to estimate your true life-line, your charted life-line, at once.

We will do this together right now, and we will start with an evaluation of your dietary balance, the number one factor of the chart. If you are still overeating—still stuffing yourself with the empty calories or sugar (and starch), you have a full strike against yourself.

If you are not on the half-portion routine, at the very least, you are trying to count yourself out, and you will not reach your 100 year plus goal. If you have not eliminated the hard fats of meat and dairy foods, you have a second strike against you. You are well on your way to becoming a food suicide.

If you have not yet begun to substitute the safe, defender fats—the polyunsaturated safflower oil type of fat—for the hard, killer fats, resign yourself to a shorter life than your natural potential calls for.

If you have a tendency to high blood pressure, and you are still salting your food heavily—perhaps even before tasting it—you are damaging your kidneys and running the risk of a still higher blood pressure. Stop at once, or add another count against yourself.

If you are on the Longevity Diet, you will be getting the highest grade protein, the best of the essential amino acids, in ocean fish. You will be getting all the vitamins and minerals you need, especially if you are supplementing your diet with a mineral-vitamin capsule or tablet. Naturally you will be supplementing in this way if you are making up for the mineral-deficient soft water in most areas.

And now we come to the second major factor of the life or death chart—obesity.

How to Shortchange Your Heart with Overweight

If you are carrying around excess pounds, you are putting an enormous extra strain on your heart. The heart is a pump, and it has to pump blood through every artery and every capillary of your body—constantly, night and day. Each pound of fat contains miles and miles of capillaries (small blood vessels), and your heart has to pump blood through every single mile of these tiny vessels. If you are carrying around extra pounds of fat, obviously you are putting an enormous extra burden on your heart. For that matter, put a ten, twenty or thirty pound weight in your pocket and try walking around with it all day long, day after day. That is what you are doing if you are ten, twenty or thirty pounds overweight. And you must add the extra burden of toting this unnecessary weight around, an extra burden on your heart. Think of the strain, the life-shortening damage you are doing to your heart if you are overweight. Are you a potential suicide? Think it over, for if you are—and if you refuse to change—you are not going to live a long life.

Now let's look at hypertension.

Is Your Blood Pressure Too High?

When did you have your blood pressure checked last? I can't do it for you during these consultations, but you should visit your family doctor soon and check your blood pressure.

If your pressure is above the normal, you must change your ways of eating at once. If you do not, and if you persist in living and eating an anti-longevity diet, you have only yourself to blame if you die young. Don't let this be your final strike, the strike that the Umpire of Life follows with, "You're out!"

Are You a Smoker?

Are you a cigarette smoker? Then know the facts. Nicotine is a deadly poison. It stands indicted as the major cause of cancer of the lung. It causes spasm of blood vessels, as you know from my own case history. Do you want to suffer the painful spasm of intermittent claudication, as I did? Do you want to suffer the borderline death-pain of angina pectoris? Do you want to shorten your life? If you do, keep smoking.

A study of 187,783 men between the ages of 50 and 69 showed

an increasing risk of coronary disease if they counted themselves out with the following Sudden Death Chart factors:

1. A high calorie diet.
2. A high total fat diet.
3. A high saturated fat diet.
4. SMOKING

Obviously, whether you die of cancer of the lung or of heart or artery disease, you are just as dead. You are a suicide, for you will have used your "license to kill" on yourself.

What About Stress?

If you are under stress to an abnormal degree—and most of us are from time to time—part of the body reaction is in terms of blood vessel spasm. Another curious fact is that *under stress your body produces more cholesterol.* We know now, as a result of recent studies on sleep at the University of Oklahoma Medical Center, that blood cholesterol levels are even raised when a sleeper dreams! It is the content of the dream that determines how high the blood cholesterol rises, and God help us if our dreams are consistently terrifying nightmares. Could this account for sudden death during sleep?

A Case of Death for a Young Doctor While Asleep

Let me tell you about a physician who died in just this way. He was only 27 when he died, and he suffered a sudden and rapidly fatal coronary thrombosis during his sleep. He never saw the next morning.

I had seen him for rectal bleeding, and had corrected his condition by injections. He was moderately hypertensive at the time, and I suggested that he would benefit from a proper diet, shorter work hours to cut down on stress, and from ridding himself of his extra weight.

Now we know that coronary artery disease and sudden heart death is very common among physicians. The doctor leads a stressful life, worrying not only about himself and his family, as we all do, but also about his many patients and their problems. If he is a surgeon, he is also under enormous life-and-death stress every time he stands at the operating table, holding his patient's life in his hands.

Our young doctor liked to eat French food. Since the secret of good French cooking is butter, butter and still more butter, he was loading himself with solid fats, with cholesterol deposits in his vital coronary arteries. And he refused to change his diet. "I'm a fatalist," he said, "and I prefer a short life and a merry one, anyhow." He got his preference shortly afterward.

The Lessons of the Young Doctor's Suicide by Food

Your pattern of living and the length of your life are not pre-determined. Don't be a fatalist. You control your own destiny to a very large degree. Get rid of your excess weight and lower your blood pressure, if it is on its way up, by following your doctor's advice. Follow the Longevity Diet pattern in all its details, and you will be getting food delicious enough for anyone. Even the French can substitute safflower oil for butter and get the same taste results without the heart and artery damage. Cut down on stress, if you possibly can, and learn to relax whenever possible.

A good rule is never to stand if you can sit, and never to sit if you can lie down. Learn the relaxation method of Section II of this book, page 186, and you will be able to use it whenever you are confronted by sudden stress.

A Word to the Ladies

If you are a woman, you have the edge over the opposite sex in many ways. I have always said that women are superior to men. They are certainly better to look at and softer to the touch. They are wiser in the earthy wisdom that counts. They are stronger, and they live longer. One of the reasons that they live longer is the pro-tection the female sex hormone seems to give them against heart attacks.

But once they get beyond the menopausal age, once they enter the change-of-life zone, they lose this protection and are just as susceptible as men are to heart and artery disease. Women should have their physician check their level of thyroid activity with the PBI (protein-bound iodine) blood test, because a low level of thyroid function is often associated with greater susceptibility to coronary disease. The lesser thyroid function seems to make the arteries more vulnerable despite the female hormones.

Do You Think You Were Born Having a Predisposition to Heart Disease?

Is there a genetic factor in heart and blood vessel disease? If there is, we have no solid evidence to prove it. There has been some talk of a dominant gene that causes special susceptibility to high cholesterol levels. But the single study that claims this (21 per cent among Jews versus 9 per cent among non-Jews) has not been confirmed. It is more likely that certain people tend to eat too much, and the wrong foods—as you have already seen in our previous consultation. Diet is the culprit in practically every case, and not fate or genes, or any predisposition.

What About Exercise?

Activity helps to lower our blood cholesterol level. I recommend walking as a most healthful, simple, and natural form of exercise. It doesn't require any apparatus and you don't have to go to a gymnasium. If you are overweight, you are probably leading a sedentary life, getting most of your exercise from lifting a full spoon or fork to your mouth three or more hours each day. Most of us neglect to exercise as we grow older. That's one of the reasons why we do grow older.

Bicycle riding is a healthful form of exercise, and it is highly recommended by a noted heart authority. But don't overdo it at the start. Go easy when you begin, and add a little more time and distance as your muscles and heart become stronger day by day.

Avoid competitive exercise, for it causes stress. This could even apply to golf if you are competing against yourself, trying to better your score each time around.

Multiple Causation

In 1951 I wrote a book for physicians called *A Handbook of Psychosomatic Medicine* in which I pointed out that there is no single cause for any disease. There are always many factors at work, and this is certainly true for heart and artery disease. There are even some people who may form so much cholesterol within their own body that they are susceptible to arterial disease even if they are on a low fat diet. So there are some cases of heart and artery disease that are not due to dietary indiscretions.

Then we must face the fact that those patients who have serious kidney disease, diabetes, poor thyroid function, high blood pressure, and who smoke excessively, are especially susceptible to atherosclerosis. They are susceptible regardless of their diet, but exceptionally so if they are firing the cholesterol bullets into their vital organs. So we see that diet is not the *only* cause of heart and artery disease, but it is certainly the major piece of our jigsaw puzzle. And don't for a moment forget obesity when you think of multiple causation—but this, of course, is again a matter of diet. We keep coming back to diet as the First Key to Longevity, your first rule of life. In the last analysis, all the other factors in the multiple causation chain are relatively minor, and I agree with those doctors who conclude that diet is virtually a *sine qua non* for atherosclerosis and atherosclerotic disease.

Blood Coagulation and What It Can Mean to You

I have one other point to emphasize before we close this consultation, and that is the fact that the high sugar diet is especially dangerous because sugar follows the acetate route to become cholesterol in your body. So please eliminate all possible sources of sugar, especially sugar and candy. And now the clincher—the fact that a high fat diet makes your blood clot faster. This clot may be the final plug in an already narrowed vessel, the final straw that breaks the coronary's back.

More Tips on Having Fun And Living Creatively For A Mentally Healthy Long Life

Now that you know more about the atherosclerosis puzzle threatening you, you have a still better chance for those 100 and more years of life. So let's see what we do to make them all good fun as well as productive and useful.

Get a hobby, if you don't already have one, and become an expert in your hobby. You might want to become a stamp or coin collector. Or you may prefer to collect sea shells or butterflies. I no longer collect things, although I did collect both stamps and coins when I was much younger. I now *collect ideas,* and you can, too. Read, underline the ideas you like best, and record them in a notebook. It will expand your horizon well beyond the ordinary, and you will become a more fully rounded person as well as a fascinating conversationalist.

Collect happy thoughts. List those too. Think about them whenever you have the time, and they will brighten your day. There is magic in thinking happy thoughts. They often bring a smile to your face, and when you smile, you will feel better.

Unhappy thoughts, gloom and doom thoughts, will make you sick. They will cause the symptoms of many diseases, acting to disturb the function of all parts of your body. The antidote for such stressful thoughts is simply to *think happy thoughts.* Learn to think positively, in terms of good health and long life. Thinking will help make it so, when combined with your Longevity Diet. Keep telling yourself that life is good, life is fun, and *let yourself* be happy. No more gloom and doom! Only fun and games from now on!

Keep life simple. Don't clutter it up with too much ambition, too much desire for material gain and material goods. After all, you already possess the greatest gift of all—life itself. *Live it.* Live it *one moment at a time,* one heartbeat at a time. Remember the wisdom of "sufficient unto the day are the cares thereof," and let tomorrow take care of itself. Enjoy today—RIGHT NOW.

And NOW, in summary . . .

1. You have been introduced to the CHART OF SUDDEN DEATH (and Slow Suicide).
2. Now you know the many interrelated factors in the heart and artery disease puzzle.
3. You know the truth about smoking, high blood pressure, stress, and all the other food suicide factors.
4. You know the many ways that excess weight kills the heart.

5. You know the many ways that smoking damages both heart and arteries.

6. You have been introduced to the truth about exercise, and how it can "kill or cure." You know what form of exercise is best, and what form is dangerous.

7. You know why women are superior to men. Forgive me, men, but this is the truth.

8. You know the multiple causation route to slow or sudden death.

9. You have been offered more tips on having fun and living creatively.

CHAPTER 9

HOW ONE PERSON LIVED
TO BE NINETY-NINE
YEARS <u>YOUNG</u>

Welcome back to my consulting room. Since we are now old friends, I want you to know that I value friendship above all else. In the practice of medicine the real reward of the physician is in the appreciation of the patient. And so, my friend, to show me your appreciation for these consultations, all I ask is that you continue to follow my advice. After all, that is not asking too much. I know it is partially selfish on my part, since I want to keep my friends alive as long as possible. But it is also largely altruistic, since it is for your own good as well. This is what I want you to do.

Please keep a chart of your weight. You do not need to make an entry more than once a week if you don't want to. If you are overweight I expect that you will see a gradual reduction of one to three pounds each week. You will do this easily as you stay on the half-portion routine, taking your natural appetite depressant Cantor Cocktail before each meal. Later, I will tell you a great deal more about shedding unwanted pounds.

I want you to be sure to eat ocean fish each day. Give up the steak and beef routine. I have been addicted to it too, so I know what it can do to you and how hard it is to let go of this old beef-eating habit. Since I realize this, don't feel too badly if you go off on a tangent occasionally with a moderate slip, lapsing into the steak or beef pattern for an occasional dinner. The occasional slip won't kill you, and it does release the pent-up desire. But always remember the golden rule of moderation, and keep those slips occasional.

I would also consider it a mark of friendship if you would stick with the six to eight glasses of water each day. And don't forget your mineral (and vitamin, if you wish) supplement if your water at home is soft.

I assume, of course, that you will continue to substitute the polyunsaturated fats for the hard fat of meat and dairy foods. Are you eating a soft margarine at home? I hope so.

I hope, also, that you have shaken the universal childhood pattern of rewarding yourself with candy or cake every time you are faced with a minor frustration. We all do it—but it is emotionally immature, and *deadly to your arteries and heart.* Please give it up, and we will both feel better about your chances for reaching 100 or more years of age.

After our eighth consultation I assume that you have given up cigarettes. I realize that this is not easy, but I have done it, and I will never ask you to do anything that I would not do. I always remember what Mark Twain said when he was asked about his smoking. "It's easy to quit smoking," he mused, "I've done it a hundred times."

I only expect you to do it once. But if smoke you must, let it be a pipe or cigars. They do not appear to cause cancer of the lung, and since you will not inhale (I hope), you will get a lesser dose of the deadly nicotine. Alright, my friend, that's what I expect from you. As an interim reward for your cooperation, I will now tell you the story of how the Longevity Diet kept a very sick man alive for 99 active, creative years—and did it over 400 years ago!

Turn Back the Aging Clock—Even after 40 Years of Age!

Everyone over 21 hears alarming stories of declining powers from that point on. And those who have reached the "failing forties" are even more resigned to loss of vitality and virility, lessening of creativity, and a relatively early feeble old age. I don't care what your age is, and I call all this resignation to premature senility the most dangerous form of nonsense.

In the first place, there is chronological age—the number of years since you were born. But there is the much more important *physiological age*—the age of your vital body tissues as represented by the way they do their work. And then there is your attitude age— the way you think about yourself. If you think you are old, you will be. If you think young, you will act young and you will become younger with each passing day. That is part of the secret of turning back the clock.

You may be in your 60's or 70's chronologically, but in your 40's physiologically. I intend to continue to show you how to do exactly that. You already know the first step, the first key, the Nutritional Key, the Longevity Diet.

You already know that nutrition is the key to easing the work of your never-resting heart. You have seen how the magical minerals of ocean fish and hard water can clear your arterial passages for a healthful, revitalizing flow of life blood to your vital tissues. You already know the secret of the Cantor Cocktail, and how to use it to maintain a proper balance between the saturated and the unsaturated fats. Put your new knowledge to work, and no matter what your present age may be you will be on your way to renewed vitality, longer life, happier living, on your way to turning back the clock.

Proof from the Astounding Case History of Luigi Cornaro

In the year 1550, Luigi Cornaro, then 83 years old, wrote his famous essay on health and longevity, in which he recommended regularity in living and simple food in small amounts. Does that sound familiar?

Cornaro was an Italian nobleman who lived from the year 1467 to 1565. *Even in that time of poor sanitation and epidemic disease, he lived to be 99 years old!* His story is particularly valuable to us because he was born with a frail constitution and very nearly died before he was 40 years of age as a result of excessive eating and drinking. His life well illustrates the value of a simple, spare diet in *reversing disease and prolonging life.*

Right there we find the tremendous importance of this story from the distant past. No matter what your present condition, serious disease can be conquered, the clock can be turned back. If it could be done 400 years ago, certainly it can be done still better today. We are living in an age of medical miracles, an age of organ transplants, artificial body parts, magnificent plastic surgery, and hormone and other medical research designed to keep us going even after nature has apparently given up. We have much to learn from Cornaro, and even more hope from the lessons of 400 years ago when transposed to today's age of medical miracles. And now I shall let Luigi Cornaro tell his own story: "O wretched and unhappy Italy! Do not you see that intemperance murders every year more of your subjects than you could lose by the most cruel plagues, or by fire and sword in many battles? Those truly shameful feasts now so much in fashion, and so intolerably profuse that no tables are large enough to hold the dishes, which renders it necessary to heap them one upon another!

"There are means still left to banish intemperance, and such means, too, that every man may have recourse to them without any assistance. Nothing more is requisite for this purpose than to live up to the simplicity dictated by nature, which teaches us to be content with little . . ., and to accustom ourselves to eat no more than is absolutely necessary to support life, considering that what exceeds this is disease and death, and merely gives the palate the satisfaction of which, though but momentary, brings on the body a long and lasting train of disagreeable sensations, and at length destroys us all."

Our mentor from the past goes on to describe his "heavy train of infirmities, including stomach disorders, gout, and almost continual low fever, and a perpetual thirst,"—a description of his condition between the ages of 35 and 40. It could well be that the continual thirst and the never-satisfied appetite represented diabetes.

How to Counteract Dissipation and Intemperance

Convinced by his physicians that he did not have long to live unless he changed to a "sober and regular life," Cornaro "resolved, in order to avoid at once both death and diseases, to betake myself to a regular course of life." By changing his dietary habits, eating simply and in small quantity, "the consequence was that in a few days I began to perceive that such a course agreed with me very well; and by pursuing it, in less than a year I found myself freed from all my complaints."

You can do the same, no matter what your present problems are (outside of cancer and the like), and the rule of moderation is your major guide to renewed health and longer life.

Cornaro's Major Lesson For You

It is most important for you to draw the major lesson of the Luigi Cornaro story right now, and to mark it well for all time. Regularity of living and a simple diet strengthened not only his body but also his mind. "Thus it is plain the neither melancholy not any other affection of the mind can hurt bodies governed with temperance and regularity. . . . Even misfortunes themselves can do but very little mischief, or cause very little pain to such bodies."

I agree completely. After you have been on the Longevity Diet and the rest of my Longevity Program for a time, you will also bear witness to your new health of body and mind. You, too, will bear witness that you can now withstand even "the slings and arrows of outrageous fortune" much better than you could before you began to turn back the aging clock.

Cornaro goes on to prove this statement by recounting financial and other misfortunes, and even an accident in which he suffered a dislocated leg and arm, from all of which he recovered rapidly and completely—*at the age of 70!*

The Cornaro Rule of Moderation

From this he concluded, "Whoever leads a sober and regular life, and commits no excess in his diet, can suffer but very little from disorders of any other kind or external accidents. On the contrary, I conclude, especially from the late trial I have had, that excess in eating and drinking are fatal."

Our wise Italian nobleman offered the very good advice that we must eat only that which agrees with us. We could all benefit from this principle. And he offers two additional "natural and very true proverbs—one, that he who has a mind to eat a great deal must eat but little . . . that eating little makes a man live very long, and living very long he must eat a great deal," and two, that "what we leave after making a hearty meal does us more good than what we have eaten."

And there, my friend, you have wisdom to which I can add nothing. Underline these words in red, and refer back to them each day before you have breakfast. They may well save your life. They will certainly add years to your life and allow you to add life to your years.

Cornaro's Simple Plan to Strengthen Both Mind and Body

The Cornaro plan of living revolved around a diet of only 12 ounces of food and 14 ounces of wine each day. On the rare occasions in which he was persuaded (against his better judgment) to increase the quantity of food, he became "peevish and melancholy, and suffered violent pain and fever." He recovered quickly from these disabilities, even in his 78th year, simply by returning to his regular limited quantity of food.

His diet included bread, meat, the yolk of an egg and soup, as well as the wine. While it is not the diet I would recommend, it apparently proves the human body is very adaptable, and that by keeping the quantity of food to the basic minimal level it is possible to prolong life.

In fact, the major lesson I want you to learn from this simple diet is the tremendous value of the limited calorie food plan. The Longevity Diet offers a great variety of foods, and I have even suggested supplementing it with a mineral (and vitamin, if you wish) capsule or tablet. But the emphasis must always be on the half-portion idea. Bear in mind that the main point is to eat as little as possible, never more than you need to reach and maintain the best weight for your age, sex, height and body build (see Table, page 144).

Always remember that half the food you eat keeps you alive and the other half kills you. The Cornaro story proves this point, as do the many hundreds of my own patients, and the entire population of the world. The trick is to eat only the half that keeps you alive, and to omit the other half altogether!

And now let's get back to the fascinating Italian sage. At the age of 86, in the year of 1553, Cornaro apparently modified his diet rules as follows: "The things I eat are: first, bread, panado (a prepared dish containing soaked bread crumbs), some broth with an egg in it, or some other good kinds of soup or spoon meat. Of flesh meat, I eat veal, kid and mutton. I eat poultry of every kind. I eat partridges and other birds, such as thrushes. I likewise eat fish, for instance, the goldney and the like amongst sea fish, and the pike and and such-like, amongst fresh water fish."

Obviously Cornaro understood the importance of individualizing any diet, but he stressed the most important rule that, "There is no necessity for eating more than the stomach can digest." That is the rule I want you to stress—the golden rule of moderation. And as the Cantor Cocktail helps you control your appetite, and as the half-portion idea helps you return your stomach to its normal size, you too will be able to live the rule of moderation just as Cornaro did 400 years ago.

Eat Less as You Reach out for the Century Mark

By the age of 95, Cornaro had found that the body needs less and less food as it grows older. He bemoaned his own genetic structure, saying, "But as I was born with feeble stamina, I am afraid I shall not outlive an hundred." But he hastened to add, with more optimism. "Were others, too, who also were born with an infirm constitution, to betake themselves to a regular life, as I have done, they would attain the age of 100 and upwards, as will be my case."

A Sound Mind in a Sound Body—at Any Age

The words *body* and *mind* are artificial separations from the facts of life. There is no such thing as a mind separate from a body, or a body without a mind (except for the imbecile). Mind and body are one, a unity. Just as urination is a function of the kidneys, the mind is simply a function of the nervous system, part of the total body function, in fact.

The importance of this realization of the unity of mind and body is that when you restore your body to more perfect health, when you revitalize your tissues, you will, at the same time, be restoring and strengthening the body function we call *mind*. Luigi Cornaro went on record that all his faculties, including good judgment, memory and spirits, were as good as ever at 95. "I find myself hearty and content, eating with a good appetite and sleeping soundly. All my faculties, at 95, are as good as ever, and in the highest perfection; my understanding is clearer and better than ever, my judgment is sound, my memory is tenacious, and my spirits are good."

You can do the same.

The Modified Cornaro Diet

It is interesting to note that the modified Cornaro diet, stressing poultry and fish, as well as a limited and truly minimal caloric intake, meets the requirements of modern research. The thinking, the principles, and the long life of Luigi Cornaro substantiate and illustrate the benefits of the modern Longevity Diet. And so we reach back over 400 years into the past to find both confirmation and inspiration. Now you know that even in those relatively primitive times, and without the benefit of modern medical knowledge or modern hygiene, it was possible to live at least 99 years. The major lesson, however, is that *it was possible to do this even when the start was made after 40 years of age*, and after dissipation almost to the point of death.

No matter what your present condition, no matter what your present age, it is not too late to begin the Longevity Diet and the total Longevity plan offered by the Four Keys to Longevity. The time for you to start is NOW. It is never too late.

The Cornaro Rules for Long Life

The fascinating story of Luigi Cornaro brings us two simple rules:

1. Eat simply, carefully, and in small quantities.
2. Regularity of living can strengthen not only your body but also your mind (the body-mind unity).*

Once you truly understand the significance of the Cornaro story

---

* Read *UNITROL: The Healing Magic of The Mind*. West Nyack, N.Y.: The Parker Publishing Co., Inc., for full details.

and of the Cornaro rules, you will no longer want to eat the large meals of your past. You will gladly reach out for the sound mind-body, the revitalized structure that will give you better mental and physical health. You will gladly turn the first Key to Longevity, the Key of Nutrition, to open the door to longer and healthier physical and mental life.

And now I want to illustrate just how *you* can do this, by telling you the story of the executive who stopped committing suicide and started to live, after he had reached a condition even worse than that of the fabled Luigi Cornaro.

The Case of the Dissipated Executive

Among the many thousands of modern counterparts of Luigi Cornaro, one patient stands out in my mind. He was an important executive "on his way up" in industry. However, he had forgotten the importance of moderation in food and drink—as well as in work. The pressures of his work, his attitudes toward that work, and his intemperance in eating and drinking were all conspiring to age him rapidly, and to terminate his life long before his natural capacity for good health and longevity might have been exhausted. He was obviously exercising his "license to kill" on himself, firing the slow bullets of stress, excess food, and drink into every vital organ of his body.

When I first saw him he was obviously under great strain, much distressed by an active "colitis." "My bowels move almost constantly," he said, "and always at the wrong time. During an important business luncheon, I will always have to excuse myself two or three times."

He often played golf with other executives in his company, and with important clients or potential customers. "When we get back to the club house, I have to settle my nerves with a few drinks." It turned out that the "few drinks" actually added up to the major part of a fifth of scotch. Sometimes he varied this by a variety of gin drinks, and always drank gin before meals and brandy afterward. "You have to keep up with the customer," he explained, "if you want to keep the customer." (The customers were all obviously would be "suicides" also!) Naturally he had to "steady his nerves" again at the end of each frustrating day. His wife joined him at that time, and they usually drank themselves into a stupor before going to bed. This was their regular routine.

A heavy drinker very often eats relatively little food. However, our budding executive was a member of the expense account set. He dined in the very finest restaurants, and did not stint on food. Each luncheon and business dinner was a veritable Roman feast of many courses. If the client wanted wine with a meal—and he usually did—he got several types, one with each course. Indeed, Mr. Executive took great pride in his knowledge of wines. "I can almost tell which side of the hill the grapes grew on," he boasted.

The combination of excessive alcohol, excessive food, late hours, the stress of business pressures, and a liberal sprinkling of "expense account girls," rivaled and in many respects exceeded the Cornaro story of youthful dissipation. And lest we forget—he smoked two packs of cigarettes each and every day.

When I examined him he had a distressing ulcerative colitis, bleeding hemorrhoids, evidence of early liver damage, and kidney disorder. Although only 41 years of age, his blood pressure was abnormally high. He had an unusually rapid pulse, and many evidences of an unstable nervous system. He was almost entirely gray, and looked well into his late 50's or early 60's, as you might expect.

His hands showed a fine tremor as he chain-smoked. The palms of his hands were always moist. A distressing habit of constantly crossing and uncrossing his legs must have been as annoying to his business associates as it was to me.

I presented the facts of the diagnosis to this patient without reservation—but kindly—as I always do. He and his wife were candidly informed that unless major changes were made in the patient's attitude, diet and drinking habits, the colitis and other conditions could not be brought under control, and his life undoubtedly would be shortened considerably.

"Frankly," I told him, "it is doubtful that you will get much further in the business world if you continue at this pace. The organization man who tries to hold too much liquor doesn't go very far or stay very long in a company as large and as important as yours."

My patient was intelligent, and he wanted to live. He had been firing the slow bullets of self-destruction for many years, but he had not realized that he was truly committing suicide. He seemed appalled at the now obvious fact.

He recognized the urgent need to change his habits—especially his drinking habits—if he was to survive. His wife was part of the drinking pattern, and although her problem was still well within control, she realized it was essential that she change at the same time. Both of them confessed that "things are in such a terrible mess" (she started to cry), "we have nothing to hold on to. Where do we start, Doctor?"

The Solution for This Dissipated Executive

It was clear to me that if this man and his wife were to be saved, they must be given a way of life that had regularity and good sense —the Cornaro way of life, the Longevity Diet way of life. It was important that they be given new hopes, a goal of good health toward which they could work. I then and there told them the inspiring story of Luigi Cornaro. Once I had convinced them that something could be done if only they had the will, I suggested my Longevity Diet to them. I also showed them the SUDDEN DEATH CHART (see previous chapter), and told them that from that point on they had it in their own power to chart their own LIFE LINE.

I stressed the enormous importance of simplicity of living, and the avoidance of unnecessary anxiety and overwork. I showed them the dangers of cigarette smoking—dangers to heart, arteries, stomach (peptic ulcer!) and to lungs.

I introduced them to simple methods of relaxation, and urged them to read and study *UNITROL: The Healing Magic of The Mind.*

Finally, I told them that if they did exactly as I said, they had a very good chance of restoring their bodies and minds to new health and greater vitality. They had a chance of living out their natural life-span—perhaps to 100 or more years.

The Healing Magic of Diet and Moderation

Slowly, ever so slowly, our old-young executive slowed down on his drinking. He learned to like the Cantor Cocktail before meals, although he considered it a poor substitute for his previous cocktails.

He began to watch his food, and the half-portion idea caught on quickly with both him and his wife. He remembered Luigi's advice to eat simply, carefully and in small quantity. He also set a regular pattern of family life that included sufficient sleep and relaxation. Most important of all, he began to enjoy the gourmet diet of our Longevity pattern—the one *you* are on right now.

As he and his wife developed more understanding, his self-control improved and his motivation to live and to be well changed his entire personality. He finally not only gave up alcohol, but also smoking. In both of these problem areas he had the moral support, example, and encouragement of a wonderful wife who was able to change her own habits as her husband changed his.

The changes in the patient's diet, combined with the necessary medications and local treatment in my office, resulted in prompt improvement in his colitis. Within a few weeks after his new diet pattern became habitual, the frequency of bowel movements decreased to a relatively normal level.

Wonder of wonders—the change in his appearance and behavior was most remarkable. He looked "ten years younger," to quote his wife. I must say the same for her. He was in much better control of his muscular and nervous systems, and his hand tremor and the uncontrolled crossing and uncrossing of his legs soon disappeared. With the decreased strain on his intestinal tract, which resulted primarily from the diet changes, his hemorrhoids shrank to negligible proportions. A few injections were used to control the bleeding from these areas, and surgery was not required.

A Person's Healthy Mind and Body Means Better Business for Him

The tremendous improvement in our problem patient's habits, appearance, and self-control had the expected effect on his business and personal relationships. Several years after his first visit to my consulting room he became the head of his company. He is now a well-respected community leader, and looks forward to many more years of happy, constructive life. When I last saw him he was "out to beat the Luigi Cornaro record of 99 years!" I believe that he might well do that, just as I hope that you also will.

More Bonuses for You with the Longevity Diet

We have emphasized the life-saving anti-coronary heart attack effect of the Longevity Diet, and you may feel that the entire story has been told. But I want you to keep in mind that there are other health bonuses to be expected. Let us return to our friend of yester-year, Luigi Cornaro, for a moment. Remember that one of the main benefits he found in his new diet was that we "can suffer but very little from disorder of any other kind." Dwell on that thought for a moment . . . it's very important. Leading nutritional studies have repeatedly found that the high calorie, saturated fat diet that is the basis of the usual American diet has been associated with a great frequency of such metabolic diseases as diabetes, gout, arthritis, and gall bladder problems.

It is certainly no mere chance that over seven out of every ten diabetic patients are found to be overweight when their symptoms first appear. On the other hand, it has been proven that only about one person in 20 is underweight when diabetes is first diagnosed. Luigi himself probably had diabetes, judging from his symptoms.

Many diabetics who are alive today and carrying on normally owe their existence to the miracle of insulin. With diabetes the body cannot burn sugar properly, and it is obvious that we should do everything possible to help the system in its proper function. Insulin cannot do its job as efficiently on a diet full of sugar as it might on the low sugar Longevity Diet—another bonus if you have this problem, or a family tendency toward diabetes.

Prevention and the A.M.A.

The Council on Foods and Nutrition of the American Medical Association has investigated the effect of fat upon a variety of medical problems, and in 1962 the Council listed "gall bladder disease" as one of the "major indications for modifying dietary fat." It appears that the proper diet will actually prevent certain types of gall stones.

Note well that important word *prevent*. I must caution you that the best treatment for aggravated cases of gall stones, once they have formed, is to remove them surgically. But for prevention, I recommend that you follow the Longevity Diet. Cut down your total fats, replace the saturated fats by the polyunsaturated oils (especially safflower oil), and limit the amount of food you eat. This is your best bet to reduce your chances of winding up on an operating table.

How Miss K Quit Being a "Fat Girl"

We have time for one more interesting problem case before closing this consultation. I want to tell you about a young lady whom we will call K, since her first name began with a K and she was well on her way to self-destruction by means of the slow bullets fired by her fattening diet.

She came from a fine family, whose home was a delight to visit. Her parents and her brother and sisters were exceptionally attractive people with groups of devoted friends. But K was shy. You see, she was more than 75 pounds overweight. While her sisters wore the latest styles and were in constant demand among the young men, our problem patient remained at home. Needless to say, this depressed her, increased her anxiety, and this in turn caused her to "reward herself" for suffering this frustration by eating box after box of candy. So the fat piled on, and the cholesterol poured into her arteries, making her old before her time. That is part of the secret psychology of obesity.

One day a former patient of mine chanced to be visiting with K, who broke down and poured out her story of unhappiness. My patient suggested that a medical consultation might be in order. I pointed out to this very bright young lady that she was literally committing suicide, and told her about the slow bullets she herself was firing every time she popped a candy into her mouth. I showed her that the fortress of fat within which she was hiding was a deadly fortress that was infiltrating her very arteries and heart. I showed her the psychological problems of the overweight frustration-complex. Being a very sensible girl, she decided to try the Longevity Diet.

Soon she began to lose weight—the required one to three pounds each week. Her mental outlook changed at once, and she became more cheerful, more extroverted, more anxious than ever to continue with her weight-losing program.

Her parents were delighted with the change and treated her to a whole new wardrobe. Once she had worn only "boxy" jackets. Now she began to appear in the latest slimming fashions. In fact, only three months later she was on her way to becoming a fashion writer. Three months after that she was to be seen modeling for one of the high fashion manufacturers.

She is now married to a very successful man (who followed his wife's example of sensible Longevity Diet eating), and is known as one of the most gracious hostesses in her city. Obviously, the psychological aspects of the Longevity Diet plan are just as important in the total revitalization process as the food itself. We will have much more to say about this secret psychology in later consultations.

More Fun Tips For Creative Living

Enthusiasm is the keynote to *fun* living. Lose your enthusiasm and you have lost all. Regain your enthusiasm and you have regained all. You will have conquered life. And so I offer you *enthusiasm therapy*. Begin each day with a smile and see how much brighter the day becomes—even if it is raining, even if there is a hurricane or an earthquake tumbling the house around. We are creatures of our emotions, our attitudes. Think enthusiasm, feel enthusiasm, and you will become a new person—full of life and vitality, the *life* of the party of *life*.

Life *is* a party. Try to enjoy it.

Your emotions control your health. I have written a whole book on this subject, 271 fully packed pages (*Ridding Yourself of Psychosomatic Health Wreckers*), but all you need to know for now is that this is a fact. Since it is a fact, you must practice happy, enthusiastic, optimistic, *positive* thinking. As you think, so will you be. Think young. Think fun. Think good luck. Think happiness. Think good health.

Your emotions are important in the control of every body tissue, all your powerful body hormones. Think good health and your tissues, your hormones, will all fall into line—into proper balance—so that your body can best restore itself to good health.

If you act with courage and determination, the world is your oyster. You can overcome truly great obstacles if you are determined to do so. Move ahead confidently, cheerfully, with the certainty that you will overcome—and you will! Seek and ye will find! Knock and it will be opened unto you!

Your subconscious mind will find the way, acting through your hormones and all other body tissues, to make your dreams come true. Nero Wolfe, the famous detective story writer, tells us that all his stories are written by his subconscious mind. Many famous inventors and creative people of all kinds tell us the same thing.

Learn to mobilize your subconscious forces and you will have learned the magic force that moves the world, your world and mine. How do you learn this magic? I show you exactly how in my other books,* and to some extent in this very set of consultations, in the Second Part of this book. The power is within you. Use it! Use it to live! Use it to work miracles!

And NOW, in summary . . .

1. We have reviewed the keys to progress—your chart for longer and happier life—*your life.*
2. Now you know that you can turn back the aging clock—become younger and healthier and happier—even if you do not start this Longevity routine until you are over 40, and even well beyond.
3. Now you know that you can turn back your aging clock even if you are suffering from chronic disease at this very moment.
4. Now you know that the Longevity Diet will help restore your body to better health, ridding you of your chronic problems while giving you new vitality and the promise of longer life.
5. Now you know the difference between chronological age and physiological age, and the important findings of *attitude-age.*
6. Speaking to you from the past, from four centuries ago, you have listened to the charm and wisdom of Luigi Cornaro, and you have learned his health and long-life secrets.
7. And you have heard the modern counterpart telling you

* Write to the UNITROL Teaching Institute, 147-41 Sanford Ave., Flushing, 11355, N.Y., for full information. Do it NOW!

how to overcome disease, dissipation and intemperance in our own day and age.

8. Now you know that both mind and body (the mind-body unity) can be restored to good health while you are shedding the effects of premature aging.

9. You have learned that you, too, can have a sound mind in a sound body—at any age.

10. You have been introduced to the healing magic of the mind and diet.

11. You have seen the many other bonuses of good health and happiness offered by the Longevity Program—*bonuses for you.*

12. You can even *prevent* gall stones (in many cases) by the proper diet.

13. The secret psychology of the Longevity Diet has been revealed to you.

14. And finally, I have given you still more tips for *fun* living.

CHAPTER 10

HOW TO JOIN THE
"ANTI-CORONARY CLUB"

Make yourself comfortable for this consultation, but don't light up a cigarette. In my waiting room you will see the request, "PLEASE DO NOT SMOKE," on every magazine table. Incidentally, did you notice that I have only recent issues of practically all the popular magazines? The no-smoking request is firmly based on the desire to keep all my patients alive as long as possible. The new magazines idea is rooted in the belief that there is very little point in staying alive if you do not keep up-to-date, if you are not aware of the passing scene, or if you take no part in the new and the different. Stay alive and *live*—RIGHT NOW. That is our objective. I assume that:

1. You are keeping your weight down and are working gradually toward the ideal longevity weight.
2. You are on the half-portion or less diet.
3. You have cut sugars and starch foods to an absolute minimum.
4. You have substituted the polyunsaturated fats for the hard and deadly fats of meat and dairy foods.
5. You are enjoying ocean fish each day.
6. You are restoring your fluid balance and your mineral requirements by hard water (or with a mineral supplement).
7. You have stopped cigarettes—not gradually—but RIGHT NOW.
8. You have learned to roll with the punches, avoiding stress where possible, and adjusting to the inevitable where necessary.

Alright, then, we are ready to move ahead with your revitalization program.

The Anti-Coronary Club

Today I want to tell you about the Anti-Coronary Club of New York and I want to invite you to join with me in forming our own personal Anti-Coronary Club. If you like the idea, just drop me a note and we will move ahead with our plans. After all, the UNITROL Teaching Institute is designed to teach us how to live as long as possible, in the best possible health, with full creative capacities released for our own advancement and for the good of all peoples. There can be no better first step than the prevention and control of coronary disease—the defeat of the number one killer, heart and artery disease. So let's set up our own Anti-Coronary Club on an international scale, with a small annual dues and membership cards, and provide the latest health information by mail for our entire membership. Do you want card number ONE? Drop me a note after this consultation, and if there is enough interest, we will go to work together to make the dream of long life and better health a reality for the entire world.

The New York Club

The Anti-Coronary Club, officially known as the Diet and Coronary Heart Disease Project, was started in New York in 1957 by the late famed nutritionist, Dr. N. Joliffe. Its purpose was to provide a public health test of the "quality-of-fat hypothesis in the etiology of coronary artery disease."

The results are now in from a four-year field study, and they prove the value of the Longevity Diet as it relates to the polyunsaturated fat versus the saturated fat idea. Naturally, we go many steps further, as you have already learned, since our objective is to prevent heart and artery disease only as the first step to long life and better general health. The New York researchers came to the conclusion that dietary control is a "feasible approach" to the reduction of coronary heart disease. That is putting it mildly, since many other studies have since confirmed and extended this conclusion.

Benefits of the Prudent Diet

A team of University of Chicago researchers showed that a "prudent" diet can help prevent atherosclerosis, today's number one killer. They did it by experiments on monkeys, since monkeys and man are very similar in body structure and function.

Over a period of two years one group of monkeys—the lucky group—was fed the "prudent diet" (low total fat, high polyunsaturated fat, just like our own Longevity Diet), while the other group of monkeys was given the "typical American" diet. And here is the heart-warming (another pun!) conclusion of these researchers: there were striking differences in the amount of fat deposited on the artery walls and in the circulating blood. This 1965 report confirms absolutely and without question everything you have learned to this point during our consultations.

Less Calories and Less Hard Fat—the Backbone of the Prudent Diet

The prudent diet—and this is the diet used by the New York Anti-Coronary Club as well—contains less calories, less cholesterol and fat, and especially less saturated fat, than does the typical American diet. The American diet is a killer—as you have already learned—firing the slow bullets of hard fat and cholesterol and calories into your vital arteries and heart. This monkey experiment is important since it is the first time that diets prepared in the kitchen and identical with those eaten by the average American, have been used to study experimental animals who develop symptoms of atherosclerosis just like those you and I might show. Take heed and take heart. Learn the lesson and live. Ignore it at your own peril.

The American Heart Association's Conclusions

A New Jersey Atherosclerosis Research Center researcher reported on a five-year study of 200 men between the ages of 20 and 50, all of whom had one or more heart attacks. The conclusion? A low-fat diet definitely cuts both recurrence and mortality rates! The treated group received a 30 per cent fat diet with added polyunsaturated fats. The nondieting group had an average 40 to 50 per cent fat diet. And there you have the proof in a nutshell. Monkeys and people react in the same way when exposed to the killer fats, or protected by the defender fats. Monkeys are indeed "the craziest people"—especially when they are "crazy" enough to commit suicide in the "people" way.

If You Are an Egg Lover

If you absolutely must have eggs, there is good news from the Cleveland Clinic, reported at the same meeting. A study on 50 "free-living normal people" on a diet in which the fat came from two servings of lean meat, fish or poultry each day, with unsaturated fat added as cottonseed oil and unsaturated margarine, was tried with one, one and a half or two whole eggs a day for 18 days.

The conclusion? Four eggs a week is a safe allowance. Use your own judgment. I prefer to play it safe and take a whole egg only as an occasional "slip," if the emotional pull is too strong to resist. My own policy is to eat only the whites of hard boiled eggs. This is high grade protein and there is no risk.

A New York City Health Department Report

A New York City Health Department report showed that when we compare those on the "prudent diet" with those people who eat the usual high fat, high caloric foods, the first group will be relatively well protected against the type of heart attacks that are practically epidemic in the second group.

There is a now-famous population study that has been going on for over 15 years at this writing, in Framingham, Massachusetts— a study of importance to all of us. These researchers showed that the middle-aged group will have coronary heart attacks at the rate of 14.5 out of every thousand. But—and here is the good news— the Anti-Coronary Club members, all in the same age group, but on a controlled low total fat, high polyunsaturated fat diet—only had 3.4 attacks per thousand! That should make you feel good, especially since you are now well started on your own Longevity Diet. Your chances of getting a coronary heart attack are now much reduced compared to before. Your chances for 100 or more years of life are much increased compared to before we met. The rest is obviously up to you.

Tobacco Statistics You Should Know

Let me give you some brief statistics, just to round out the story, and then I will tell you about one of my patients who gave up smoking just in time to save his life.

Cigarette smokers who smoke two packs a day or more, suffer sudden death from heart attacks five times more often than non-smokers. Smokers also have twice as many attacks of heart muscle destruction and twice as many complaints of angina pectoris (heart pain). Let me quote the researchers: "In short, a person with high blood pressure, cholesterol, or electrocardiogram abnormalities is sicker with smoking."

How the Longevity Diet Helped John in Quitting the Cigarette Habit

John, a troublesome and almost suicidal patient, was only 27 years old. He was a crackerjack mechanic, and he smoked a deadly two packs of cigarettes each day. Despite his youth, he already had all the evidences of angina pectoris. "I get pain in my chest every time I do a little extra work. Lately I even get it when I am sitting down, especially after a heavy meal." His blood cholesterol level was high, and he also had a third strike in an elevated blood pressure.

I gave him the facts straight, and he didn't flinch. But he did nothing about it. "I *need* cigarettes," he whined. "I have to have them."

"You need them about as much as you need a hole in your heart," I told him. But he continued to smoke.

One day he almost paid the final price. He had a coronary closure that put him to bed for two weeks, and kept him from work for two additional weeks after he left his bed. Fortunately there was no serious heart muscle damage. That raised the red flag for him, and saved his life. He stopped smoking. He also meekly and wisely accepted the Longevity Diet. The result?

His blood pressure returned to normal. His blood cholesterol came back to normal. His angina pectoris pain stopped. He could work "round the clock" without chest pain and without fear of sudden death. His Longevity Diet was his "ace" in kicking the cigarette habit.

Physical Activity And Your Heart

Famed Harvard nutritionist, Dr. Frederick J. Stare, tells us that recent results in a study of 700 Boston Irishmen compared with their brothers who stayed in Ireland showed that "activity is the key to cardiac (heart) well-being." The Boston group—30 to 60 years of age—suffered coronary disease heart deaths in twice as many cases as their counterparts in Ireland. This was in spite of the fact that the Ireland men ate more eggs, more butter, and more of the other saturated fats (but had *lower* blood cholesterol levels!). This proves the enormous value of activity—normal exercise with work—in lowering the blood cholesterol level and preventing heart attacks.

Tobacco and Calories Hasten Death

But there were other factors. For example, the Boston Irishmen smoked more than their brothers in the "old country." As to calories, exercise can even overcome a certain excess of food. This was proven by the fact that the men of Ireland ate 400 more calories per day than their Boston brothers, *but weighed 10 per cent less.* Obviously the men of Ireland were getting more exercise, and their lower cholesterol levels proved that this physical activity burned off the excess calories and lowered the blood cholesterol.

How Mary Used Exercise to Lower Her Weight

Mary loved to lie in bed until the late hours of the morning, and to lie down and watch television during the afternoon hours, while munching on chocolates. She was married to an indulgent husband who did not seem to mind his wife's habits or her rapidly increasing weight. He himself was quite slim, since he ate little and worked hard as a bus driver. I do not know what their apartment looked like, since Mary could not afford a maid, and certainly must have done little or nothing to keep it clean.

At 41 she was twice the size she should have been, had a marked elevation of blood pressure, complained of frequent headaches (due to the high blood pressure!), and was so severely constipated that I had to remove the impaction under anesthesia in my office. Her blood cholesterol level was very high, and I advised her that she would have to change her eating habits *and* her degree of general activity if she wished to stay alive.

She agreed, and did change by rising early in the morning and taking a one hour walk—rain or shine. She learned to like this morning walk, and soon added an afternoon walk as well. I rechecked her blood cholesterol level one month later, not expecting much of a change, since her weight had remained practically constant, but she surprised me by showing a good decrease in her cholesterol. This was obviously due to the exercise, since she admitted that she was still gorging herself on chocolates, and had not made the other changes required by the Longevity Diet.

It would seem that perhaps sugar is not the great villain we might think, except in terms of calories, and perhaps only to a lesser degree in terms of blood cholesterol. However, her blood pressure remained too high, and I once again cautioned her on the suicidal direction of her behavior.

She was intelligent enough to listen to reason, and began to follow the Longevity Diet pattern. Her weight loss was about two to three pounds each week, and she soon became fascinated by her new figure and more youthful face. This kept her on the right track, and she reached the optimal weight level (see page 144) within the next six months. Her blood pressure returned to normal, and her headaches stopped. Her constipation also came under control, helped by the water and vegetables in the Longevity Diet. Her suicide by food pattern had been stopped!

Risk Factors You Should Know About

A recent study gives us three diet-related risk factors as to our health. These are (1) a cholesterol blood level over 260 mg. per cent (260 mg. per hundred cc. of blood), (2) a diastolic * blood pressure of 95 mm. mercury or more, and (3) obesity.

The lady I just told you about had all three of these risk factors—three strikes against her. But she was not counted out—AND YOU NEED NOT BE COUNTED OUT, UNLESS YOU DO IT YOUR-SELF. Your fate is in your own hands, and I hope you will not choose to exercise your license to kill by aiming the deadly slow bullets against your own vital organs.

You must watch both your diet and your weight. Weight is your best guide to calories, and if you are overweight, you are simply eating too much.

Coronary Artery Disease as the SEDENTARY Disease

I consider coronary artery disease as a SEDENTARY DISEASE, and want to show you how to find the key causative elements in the word itself:

S	Stress
E	Emotions
D	Diet
E	Exercise (deficiency or competitive)
N	Neuro-psychic
T	Tobacco
A	Anxiety
R	Relaxation Resistance
Y	You (your genetic structure)

We have already gone over most of these important SUICIDE CHART factors, but I want to tell you a little more about the stress factor. It acts in several ways to damage your heart and arteries:

1. When in distress, your blood cholesterol level tends to go up.
2. Under stress, your adrenal glands pour adrenaline into your blood stream, and this raises your blood pressure and increases your heart rate.
3. Many of your blood vessels tend to contract during stress, decreasing the blood flow to your tissues.
4. Chemical changes take place both in your blood stream and in your tissues. Dr. Selye, to whom I introduced you in a previous consul-

---
* Pressure in the blood vessels.

tation, showed us that during stress there are changes in the mineral elements of the blood stream, changes that predispose our body to death of the heart muscle.

Rest Versus Exercise

I may seem to be contradicting myself when I tell you to get enough rest, and to learn how to relax, and then turn about and tell you to be active. But this is not so. You can be active while relaxed, for relaxation is largely a state of mind. I have gone into this at great length in my book, *UNITROL; The Healing Magic of The Mind,* and in *Ridding Yourself of Psychosomatic Health Wreckers.* In fact, you must learn how to be relaxed at all times if you are to avoid stress reactions of the type just described, stress that will strike you many times each day whenever you are faced by everyday annoyance and frustration.

You can be fully relaxed while walking or riding a bicycle, and yet you will be burning up the calories and lowering your blood cholesterol during this relaxing activity.

How to Relax and Exercise in Bed

Many of my patients like to relax in bed at night, and watch television for an hour or two before drifting off to sleep. And yet, when they follow my instructions, they are tightening and relaxing their leg and arm and abdominal muscles all during this period of relaxation—getting active muscle exercise while relaxing at the same time. The combination helps them sleep by tiring their body muscles by these contractions—often in time to the music of the commercials—and by tiring their eye muscles by watching television. The poor quality of the average television show is enough to tire the brain at the same time, and the combined "tired relaxation" hastens sleep, after having burned calories and lowered blood cholesterol. A wonderful combination!

The Happy Heart

The "cure" for negative thinking—for fear, anxiety, stress of all types—is obviously to change to positive, affirmative thinking and attitudes while trying with might and main to solve your problems.

A happy attitude gives us a happy heart. A happy attitude will often counteract even a dangerous diet.

This is one of the reasons why I have been concluding each of our consultations by telling you how to have fun and enjoy life. The major importance of stress and emotional disturbance in heart attacks seems to be demonstrated by a recent report from Roseto, Pennsylvania. This little town is about 110 miles from New York City, and is composed of people of Italian descent who love prosciutto ham with an inch of fat on it, fried peppers, and bread dipped in lard gravy, with plenty of Chianti to wash it all down. A "ton" of slow bullets, as you can imagine. Not only that, they are fat, hard-working and happy people. It is said that they are "without a care for tomorrow." In spite of this dangerous diet, these happy people of Italian descent do not often die of heart attacks.

In fact, a report in one of the leading medical journals on the town of Roseto showed that they had one quarter to one third the heart attack rate of a neighboring town. To make it even more remarkable, these men and women are overweight, especially the older men who are up to 80 pounds above the national average. Still worse—the daily caloric intake is 3,000 for men and 2,300 for the women, again far above the national average. Still on the debit side—most of these calories come from the deadly animal fat!

This is a puzzler, a miracle town, *contradicting everything taught by our leading nutritionists*. What is the explanation?

Answers to the Roseto Diet Puzzler

In my opinion the answers to this riddle are to be found in the way these people think and act. There is no emotional stress in this town—eliminating a major killer factor from our SUICIDE CHART. These people have learned how to enjoy life. They are gay, boisterous, and unpretentious. The wealthy dress and behave just like their less fortunate neighbors.

They are described as "simple, warm and very hospitable." There is said to be no crime in Roseto. The people are mutually trusting and mutually supporting. There is no real want since, in emergencies, neighbors provide for each other's needs. This is a self-contained and *working* anti-poverty program.

And there we have the major answer—the absence of anxiety and stress, the presence of simplicity, happiness and an active life in which men and women work even when they don't need the money.

Eliminate stress and keep active, and you will be able to lower *your* blood cholesterol and reduce the chance of a fatal heart attack, even while on a dangerous diet. But since you and I do not live in Roseto, you must stay on your Longevity Diet at the same time that you add fun and activity to your life. Besides, even if you wanted to move to Roseto, you would still take your troubled mind and wrong attitudes with you. And by the time you read this book, the younger people of Roseto will have left to join the stress- and anxiety-ridden "outer world" that you and I live in every day of our lives. The older inhabitants will live out their lives. And so we come to the ultimate realization that we must each find our own Roseto within our own mind and heart. These consultations will teach you how to locate the mythical Shangri-La, how to drink from the Fountain of Youth—for you will find these only within yourselves.

The Anti-Coronary Club Diet

The time has come to compare the New York City Anti-Coronary Club diet with our own Longevity Diet. Their "prudent diet" fat content is lowered from the usual 40 per cent of the average American diet to 30 per cent of a total diet of about 2,700 calories. One third of this fat is polyunsaturated, one third monounsaturated and the rest saturated.

Our own Longevity Diet has a lower total fat content, since I recommend 20 per cent, and a relatively much higher polyunsaturated fat content. The patient drinking the Cantor Cocktail before each meal, eating sea food daily, and reducing the amount of fatty beef in his diet, would probably be taking about two-thirds of his total fat in the polyunsaturated form. If he were on a vegetarian diet, he would be getting even more polyunsaturated fat and even less of the saturated killer fat. Total calories naturally will vary with the individual, his work, and many other factors—especially his weight. I advise a low calorie diet, as you very well know, and recommend that you let your weight be your guide. If you are overweight and not losing, you are still eating too much. You must cut down the calories—and you need count only pounds, not calories.

We can reasonably expect, therefore, that our own Longevity Diet will give us even better results than the "prudent diet" of the New York Anti-Coronary Club.

But note this. The overweight members of the Anti-Coronary Club were given a diet averaging 1,600 calories, and containing only 19 per cent of these calories as fat. This compares very favorably with our own Longevity Diet.

Anti-Coronary Club Diet Details

The New York City group is told to avoid butter, cream, ice cream, hard cheese, cream cheese, and animal fat. I agree. They are told to use vegetable oil for cooking and for salad dressing. I agree. They are told to take veal and poultry in limited amounts, but are restricted on beef, pork, lamb and mutton to only 16 ounces per week. That is a good rule.

You will be interested to know that the average member of the Club had the greatest difficulty giving up rich pastries, ice cream and large meat portions. For that matter, I had trouble, too, with ice cream and steak—two of my favorites in my former "sick" days, my "Mister Five by Five" days. And yet this group consisted primarily of well educated, health-conscious men in professional and managerial occupations. Habit and emotion are strong pressures, and even intelligent men and women who are anxious to stay alive may have difficulty in giving up their "candy and cake."

The Prudent Diet and Blood Cholesterol

You will be pleased to know some of the impressive statistics on the prudent diet results, since they are very like my own patients' results.

Here are the dry but life-saving statistics. The average cholesterol level of the first 400 men, in the 50 to 59 age group, who began this study-club was 216 mg. per 100 cc of blood. Less than 8 per cent had levels under 200 mg. per cent, and about 20 per cent of the group had blood levels under 220 mg. per 100 cc of blood.

What did the "prudent diet" do? It lowered the serum cholesterol level in about 80 per cent of the men in the highest third of the group. It did very well also for those who were fatties, bringing the cholesterol level down from 261 to 225 in over half of this group, and doing it after only six weeks on the diet.

Please remember that our goal on the Longevity Diet is to get as close to the 150 mg. per cent level as we can. That is the level that separates the "men from the boys," the level that sparates the mortality "statistics" from the 100 year or more "lucky ones." To get into this long-living group you must follow all the rules of the Longevity pattern, including the diet.

And Now for More Fun and Games

This consultation has proved to you that you must change your ways of thinking—your attitudes toward life—if you are to stay alive for 100 or more years. Remember Roseto! You must learn to *be cheerful,* even *gay* at all times. You must learn to live a *simple life.* If you are content with what you have and keep life simple, you will have the peace of mind that keeps your arteries relaxed and your blood cholesterol down.

You must learn to *love one another.* This is an important Biblical admonition, and it will work for you all the time. Remember Roseto! When you help your neighbor over the hurdles, you help yourself at the same time.

Learn to *take life as it comes.* There are some things you cannot change. Learn to adjust to those, but strive mightily to change for the better as you go along.

Learn to *think happy thoughts,* and to enjoy life each day. DANCE whenever you can. This is a new one for you. Dance at parties, in dance halls, at home in front of your radio or record player or television—whenever and wherever you can. This is one of the best forms of exercise. It makes you happy, limbers up your muscles and joints, gets rid of excess calories, and lowers your blood cholesterol. How's that for good medicine while enjoying life!

Be warm and hospitable at all times. When you give of yourself, the "bread cast upon the waters" comes back to you many times over. This is "bread" you can "eat," for it is the "bread" of life, the "bread" of love, the "bread" of human kindness and warmth.

And NOW, in summary ...

1. We have reviewed your personal progress, and I hope you are pleased with what you have done to move along the road to better health and longer life.

2. I have told you the fascinating facts about the New York Anti-Coronary Club and I have invited you to join with me in forming our own Anti-Coronary Club, an International Anti-Coronary Club.

3. I have told you the results of the New York Anti-Coronary Club diet, and have shown you how our Longevity Diet may be even better for you.

4. I have shown you the confirming studies from Chicago and other parts of the country—studies on monkey and man.

5. Now you know that the typical American diet is a killer, and that the Longevity Diet is a life-saver.

6. Now you have still more proof that cigarettes are slow bullets. Give up cigarettes and you have an enormously better chance of avoiding heart and artery disease.

7. Now you have the life-saving facts on exercise, and you know exactly how to exercise to save your own life.

8. You have been shown the various ways in which STRESS can count you out.

9. You have been shown the SEDENTARY factors of coronary heart disease.

10. I have introduced you to a method for relaxed exercising even while in bed.

11. You have met the people of Roseto and learned about the "happy heart."

12. I have once again showed you how to have more fun and how to get more out of life.

CHAPTER 11

HOW TO MAKE YOUR BASIC DIET PATTERN SIMPLE AND EFFECTIVE

Before we consider the basic diet—the essentials for your good health and long life—let us review for a moment or two all the essentials of the previous consultations. I want to be sure—since your life depends upon it—that you really understand and *are using* all the essential information of our previous talks together.

So settle back comfortably, and think back to what has been discussed in this book to date.

1. You are drinking your Cantor Cocktail before each meal, and you are now enjoying it as a delicious and healthful drink. It is more and more evident to you that the French are right when they say that "it is habit that forms our taste." Once you get into the habit of your new eating patterns, you learn to enjoy them. The foods taste good to you. That is the way it is all over the world. We have learned to enjoy whatever we have been carefully taught to expect to enjoy. Perhaps you have learned to enjoy snails and frogs legs and—yes, even olives! (I did.)

2. You have learned to look with alarm at the beef and steak staples of the American diet.

3. You have learned to enjoy fish each day.

4. You look forward to all forms of non-competitive exercise, especially dancing.

5. You now even "dance" as exercise in bed—keeping time to radio,

television or record player by contracting and relaxing various muscle groups, all without bending a joint or disturbing your bed covers.

6. You are enjoying daily long walks.

7. You are learning to cope with stress, and are becoming one of the "happy heart" people.

8. You are keeping life simple, enjoying it one moment at a time. You understand the meaning of:

Inch time
Foot gem.

Good for you! You are really on your way to better health and longer life. It is my pleasure to walk along with you, to guide you every step of the way. As you read and reread, as you understand and apply this book—these consultations in print—you will find me with you every moment of the day. And I will bring you the better health and the longer life you desire each moment of each day throughout the 365 days of each year.

There Is No Single Diet Pattern Essential for Life and Health

We are now ready to consider the basic diet. All nutritionists agree that there is no single diet pattern and no single food essential for health and life. That is an important statement, and should help you to give up all fad diets once and for all. From this point on you do not have to be bound to any single food or any single combination of foods, no matter who recommends them as the *only way* to better health. There are many ways, and I want you to understand the principles so you can choose your own way—the way you like best, the one that suits your own temperament and your own needs.

The Essentials of a Diet Program

Although our body requires a certain amount of calories to maintain itself in good repair and for energy, you know now that too many calories are dangerous, and may even be deadly. Keep to the minimum intake always.

You know now that certain fatty acids are essential for proper function, and that too much of the saturated fats can damage your arteries, shut off the blood supply to your heart, and literally kill you. You are now aware that proteins supply the essential amino acids, and that you cannot live without them, but that if these amino acids are associated with the saturated killer fats—as they are in steak, beef, pork, and so on—you have obviously looked in the wrong place for your essential protein. You should be getting your essential amino acids more safely—in fish and other foods which contain the polyunsaturated defender fats.

You now know about the miracle minerals, and how important they are to your arteries and your total body. And you certainly have had the importance of vitamins dinned into you from all directions since your earliest years. But did you know that it doesn't take much food of the right kind to provide these essential minerals and vitamins? Remember the consultation on the ancient oceans and the magic minerals? See Chapter 3, if you don't remember. I don't mind if you take a mineral supplement or even a vitamin and mineral supplement, if you wish. It can do no harm in moderation, especially if your water is the demineralized soft water.

What I am saying, in brief, is that you not only need the essential elements of a good diet, but you need to get them from the right foods if you wish to avoid trouble. And you need to practice moderation, since too much of a good thing may be deadly. Now let me take a moment to introduce you to one of my patients who thought that if a small amount was good, a larger amount would be better.

Case History: Too Much of A Good Thing May Injure You

This patient, a woman in her thirties, had lost her appetite, was often nauseated and vomited, and suffered a severe diarrhea. It developed that she had been taking very large doses of vitamin D, since she had "heard somewhere" that this was a good treatment for psoriasis (a scaly skin condition on her elbows and elsewhere). She had been taking over 100,000 international units of this "essential" vitamin each day for several months. Now she was suffering from a vitamin D overdose, and it was poisoning her.

Now vitamin D is essential for the growing child, but adults probably do not need to supplement their diet with this vitamin. It may be that some skin specialists would recommend vitamin D for the treatment of psoriasis, but the dosage would be carefully supervised by that physician.

For that matter, even in children too much vitamin D can be dangerous and damaging. Calcium may even leave the bones and be deposited in the heart, the large blood vessels, lungs, kidneys and other soft tissues.

Fortunately, this is reversible if the vitamin D is stopped in time. My patient was poisoning herself with an "essential" vitamin. When she learned the cause of her trouble, she stopped the vitamin D and was soon well. Too much of a good thing, even an *essential* food, can be dangerous. That is the lesson you must learn.

What is an Adequate Diet?

This leads us right into the question of what is an adequate diet. Obviously, we must be careful to avoid excess, even of the essential food elements. Obviously, we must be careful to avoid eating too much of *anything*—we have to restrict our intake of calories. Obviously, we must be careful to include the "right" fats, the right amino acids (proteins), the right minerals and vitamins in the right amounts, and to avoid the empty calorie sugars.

Everything I have taught you to this point, everything you have learned during our consultations, shows you that we cannot be certain that what is best for growing tall, growing up early, or for those much-admired big, strong muscles, is at the same time best for the longest life-span. As a matter of fact, if you think back to your visit with the famed Dr. McCay at Cornell (see Chapter 1) you will recall that retarded growth—an "inadequate" allowance of calories—was his key to revitalization, internal rejuvenation, and longevity.

His experiments proved that there is a definite relationship between the number of calories you take (the amount and kind of food you eat) and the diseases you suffer from and how soon you will die.

So from the point of view of better health and longer life there seems to be little question that an adequate diet is one with a minimum of food and calories. Ponder that before we move on.

I will turn it around for you—the more you eat, the sooner you will die. Now think about that.

How Can You Know How Much to Eat?

Take a look at the table of optimal weights. Let that be your guide to how much to eat. How? Simple, really. If you are over-

DESIRABLE WEIGHTS FOR MEN
of ages 25 and over

Weight in Pounds According to Frame (In Indoor Clothing)

Height (With shoes on— 1-inch heels) Feet	Inches	*Small* *Frame*	*Medium* *Frame*	*Large* *Frame*
5	2	112-120	118-129	126-141
5	3	115-123	121-133	129-144
5	4	118-126	124-136	132-148
5	5	121-129	127-139	135-152
5	6	124-133	130-143	138-156
5	7	128-137	134-147	142-161
5	8	132-141	138-152	147-166
5	9	136-145	142-156	151-170
5	10	140-150	146-160	155-174
5	11	144-154	150-165	159-179
6	0	148-158	154-170	164-184
6	1	152-162	158-175	168-189
6	2	156-167	162-180	173-194
6	3	160-171	167-185	178-199
6	4	164-175	172-190	182-204

DESIRABLE WEIGHTS FOR WOMEN
of ages 25 and over

Height (With shoes on— 2-inch heels) Feet	Inches	*Small* *Frame*	*Medium* *Frame*	*Large* *Frame*
4	10	92-98	96-107	104-119
4	11	94-101	98-110	106-122
5	0	96-104	101-113	109-125
5	1	99-107	104-116	112-128
5	2	102-110	107-119	115-131
5	3	105-113	110-122	118-134
5	4	108-116	113-126	121-138
5	5	111-119	116-130	125-142
5	6	114-123	120-135	129-146
5	7	118-127	124-139	133-150
5	8	122-131	128-143	137-154
5	9	126-135	132-147	141-158
5	10	130-140	136-151	145-163
5	11	134-144	140-155	149-168
6	0	138-148	144-159	153-173

For girls between 18 and 25, subtract 1 pound for each year under 25.

weight in terms of your height, body structure and sex, you are obviously eating too much. In other words, let your weight be your guide to how many calories you need and then simply follow the principles of the Longevity Diet to get the right kind of calories from the right kind of foods.

Your Weight-Diet Guide

From now on this table will be your weight-diet guide. I would suggest that you refer to it for each member of your family and set them all on the right path—the path to better health and longer life.

Stay on the Longevity Diet, and since it is low in calories, if you are overweight your new eating habits will bring your weight to the "normal" level, within the range shown by the table. This table is based upon the actuarial findings of the major United States insurance companies, and shows us that the average person is overweight.

Calorie Calculations

For those of you who want to calculate calories I have no objection. You may want to refer back to the consultation in Chapter 6 for the information you need on calories. You will be reminded that you don't need to count calories, but that calories do count. You will recall what a calorie is—a unit of heat energy—and how many the average person needs. You will also see again how many calories there are in the basic foods—protein (4.1 per gram), carbohydrate (4.1 per gram) and fat (9.3) per gram.

You will be reminded that the work you do is important in determining how much food you should eat. If you drive a truck you will obviously need more than if you sit at a desk and calculate figures or pound a typewriter.

But, in all cases, you had better be careful how you get those calories, what foods you choose to nourish your body and to provide the work energy you need.

How to Make Weight-Calorie Calculations

For quick calculation of your calorie requirement, based on the weight table, simply multiply each pound of your ideal body weight by 18 calories, if you are a female, and by 21 calories if you are a man. I would suggest that you modify this with a range of 15 if you do very little work, and up to 25 if you do hard physical work.

Simple enough? Yes, but again I want you to remember that if you are overweight you are probably eating too much, regardless of which figure you come up with. Bring your weight down if you really want to stay alive for that 100 or more goal.

Sugar and Starch to be Eliminated Promptly from Your Diet

My Longevity Diet advises you to virtually eliminate sugar and starch foods. An excellent clinical textbook advises us: "There is no specific requirement for carbohydrates and there is no requirement for any specific carbohydrate." Naturally, I agree.

But what if you are not overweight? If you are well under the optimal weight table level, my advice to you, if you are not feeling ill, and if your general physical examination shows no problems, is to stay underweight.

But, if you still want to put on more weight, or if your physician says you should, all you have to do is to include potatoes and the whole grain cereals in your diet. Potatoes have a high vitamin C and nicotinic acid content, and the whole grain cereals are a good source of proteins and many water-soluble vitamins.

Moderation Is Your Working Key to Successful Dieting

Your key to long life should be, "Moderation under all circumstances"—whether you are thin or heavy, tall or short, manual, office, or professional worker. For example, if you are underweight and feel you must have potatoes or whole grain cereals, I still recommend half portions. If I have the urge to eat a potato, I take it baked in the skin, and I then eat only the (well scrubbed) skin and the little layer of potato that sticks to it. I leave the rest in order to keep my weight at the optimal level. (You see, I am the kind of doctor who says, *"Do as I do."*)

If you must have a whole grain cereal for breakfast, take only half a bowl, even though it is rich in good proteins and the B and C vitamins. Always remember the ever-present and always threatening excess calories. Let moderation be your guide, your key to longer life and better health.

The Case of the Overweight Office Worker

Now let me introduce you to a very fine young man in his early twenties, a very hard working and ambitious clerk, who "grabs his meals" at a lunch counter in the financial district. He "fortifies himself" with the All-American Killer Breakfast of ham and eggs, orange juice and two cups of coffee, before leaving for work. Dinner is usually a "good steak" and potatoes (fried, of course), and pie a la mode (two scoops of ice cream), with another two or even three cups of coffee.

You could easily answer his question—"What's so bad about that?" You could answer it even more easily when you referred to the weight table and found that your new friend is over 30 pounds beyond his optimal weight. And you could emphasize your answer still better if you could watch his blood pressure readings—well into the danger zone. The blood cholesterol level confirmed the fact that he was on his way to an early coronary death if he did not change his ways.

What were his complaints? He tired easily, and so would you if you were carrying around 30 extra and heart-exhausting pounds. He had frequent headaches, and so would you if your blood pressure was over 200 at the heart level. He had "heartburn after eating," and so would you if your stomach kept pouring out excess acid on its way to burning the hole of peptic ulcer in your stomach lining.

I put him on the low calorie, low total fat Longevity Diet, and was pleased to see him go back to normal within the next six months. His weight reduction was at the ideal rate of three pounds per average week. His blood pressure and his blood cholesterol came steadily down. His heartburn disappeared and he never developed an ulcer. He regained his normal vigor and vitality, and went on to become an important executive in his firm. And he's liable to live for more than his "three score and ten."

How Much Fat Is Allowed in a Basic Diet?

I have already answered this question in several of our chapter consultations. But I want to emphasize the right answer for you, so you will not need to worry about fats. First, drink your Cantor Cocktail before each meal. If you don't get another bit of fat, that cocktail would be enough. I want you to keep your total fat foods to an absolute minimum, and certainly no more than 20 to 25 per cent of your total calories should be in the form of fat.

To accomplish this, try to avoid the "killer" fats altogether. Stay away from meat and dairy foods, except those you will find on your Longevity Diet (next chapter consultation).

When you eat your two large, mixed green vegetable salads— one as your first course at lunch and one as your first course at dinner—use safflower oil and vinegar, or safflower oil and lemon juice (and add a touch of garlic if you like), as your salad dressing. This will give you still more of the defender fats.

How Much Protein for the Basic Diet?

The National Research Council tells us that a daily protein allowance of one gram for every 2.2 pounds of body weight is required by adults. Actually there is a protein loss in daily living which must also be compensated for, amounting to about one ounce a day for the average adult. In all, then, we can say that you will probably need about two ounces of protein each day. This is not very much, and you must stay as close as possible to this minimal amount if you want to stay in the best possible health. Anything you eat above the amount that you actually need, has to be put through your body metabolism, burned up, or converted to fat—all useless and energy-consuming activities.

Now let's translate this requirement into actual food—the type that is readily available and acceptable to our Longevity Diet principles. A three-ounce can of sardines (the fabulous herring family), will give you about 25.7 grams of protein toward the daily requirement of 70 grams (about 2 ounces). A baked bluefish would give you about 27.4 grams of protein. The whites of two hard boiled eggs will provide 21.6 grams of protein.

This means that if you eat two hard boiled egg whites for breakfast, a tin of sardines for lunch, and then had a bluefish for dinner, you would have more than enough protein. And you must remember that the amount of skimmed milk you will be drinking in your three Cantor Cocktails each day will give you about 10.5 additional grams of protein.

And now for those who will occasionally slip in the direction of beef and steak, let's see where this leads us in terms of protein. It only takes about three ounces of porterhouse steak, for example, to give you 23 grams of protein. This means that if you eat a nine-ounce steak (and that isn't any more than the average steak house portion), you will be getting all the protein you need for the day. Once again you have to add your Cantor Cocktail protein to that (the protein in the skimmed milk)—10.5 grams. That isn't too bad, but think of the 81 grams of saturated fat in that nine-ounce steak— all killer fat!

A nine-ounce rib roast will give you a little more protein and a little less fat—but all of the fat will be of the killer variety.

What Kind of Protein to Eat for Best Results

The Longevity Diet is a modified vegetarian diet, and that means that much of your protein will be *vegetable protein*. However, since it is also important to have animal protein in your diet, I have included fish each day, the whites of hard boiled eggs, and skimmed milk and cottage cheese.

Fish contains a very high grade of biological protein, and also has the bonus of a high level of polyunsaturated fats. Once again I want to remind you of the special value of the herring family (including sardines) for their vanadium—one of the magical minerals.

Be Sure and Not Sorry about High Protein Foods

Let me caution you about the so-called high protein foods. I have recommended the whites of hard boiled eggs as an excellent source of animal protein. But if you eat the yolks as well, you will be getting saturated fat and cholesterol along with your protein. The same applies to beef and steak, as you have already seen. Ordinary hamburgers—the usual kind "grabbed" for lunch or dinner by most office workers and by the youngsters at all times of the day—are mostly saturated fat (three-quarters of the calories are fat calories). These are the killer fats, and that is a high price to pay for a relatively small amount of protein.

So be careful where you get your fats from, where your proteins come from, and the type of protein and fat you are eating. In a nutshell—stick to the Longevity Diet recommendations and you won't have to worry about all these little details.

The Case of the Careless Hamburger Eater

A patient was given the Longevity Diet when he came in for a postoperative checkup (hemorrhoids), and I saw that he had gained many pounds and looked many years older than his "chronological" 51. He was old before his time, and his rising blood pressure went along with his obesity and his excess weight. I checked his blood cholesterol and found it much elevated— in the 300 range.

One month later, when I rechecked him, although his weight was coming down, his cholesterol level was not. It appeared that he had drawn his own conclusions about the diet, and decided that it was simply a "high protein diet," so he chose his own protein in the form of hamburgers. "I love them," he told me. "They give me the protein you want me to have."

How wrong he was. He was killing himself with the saturated fat and the bun calories. I set him straight on the nature of hamburgers and the truth about proteins.

Six months later, after sticking strictly to the Longevity Diet, he was back to his former body size, a normal blood pressure, and his blood cholesterol was coming down from the danger zone.

Vitamins and Your Longevity Diet

The Longevity Diet will provide you with all the vitamins you need. However, if you want more, I have no objection to any vitamin or vitamin-mineral preparation your physician may advise. Many of my patients ask me about brewer's yeast. It is an excellent source of the B vitamins. But you will get the B vitamins in heart, liver, kidney (organ meats). These organ meats are not generally dangerous, for they are actually low in fat content. Chicken liver, for example, contains about 4 per cent fat, only 1 per cent of which is saturated. Beef liver is about 3 per cent fat, and again only 1 per cent is saturated. Calves liver runs higher, however—about 5 per cent fat, 2 per cent of which is saturated. To really get the saturated fats in your diet down to the minimum, you would have to avoid all animal meat, and stick to ocean fish for most of your protein and fat sources.

Wheat germ is another good food supplement to give you the B vitamins and vitamin E as well as high quality protein and iron. I often add it to my Cantor Cocktail, although it sinks to the bottom after it is blended unless you drink it promptly.

The Modified Vegetarian Diet

I want to make it clear that I do not expect you to be a strict vegetarian (although I do not object if you already are). My own recommendation is for the *lacto-ovarian (partial) vegetarian diet.* The whites of eggs offer a high grade animal protein. Skimmed milk and the cottage cheese provide other sources of animal protein of a high biological quality. I also advise ocean fish daily (and meat occasionally for those who "want" it). You can go all the way as a vegetarian by omitting all meat and fish if you wish. But since fish contains not only a very high grade biological protein, but also a high level of the life-saving polyunsaturated fatty acids, and since ocean fish gives you the magic minerals—especially vanadium—I advise you to eat fish several times each week, and preferably daily.

Food Supplements in General

Clive McCay, whom you met in his Cornell University laboratory, advises that you keep a sugar bowl on your table filled with powdered bone meal and another filled with wheat germ, to eat at each meal. He also reminds us that brewer's yeast is one of the richest natural sources of both protein and water soluble vitamins. Listen to McCay: "It can be taken suspended in water just before meals by those who tend to become overweight. It can be used to lessen the need for insulin by diabetics. It may help prevent constipation."

As you already know, I have no objection to any of these natural food supplements, since they are very good sources of vitamins, protein, and minerals. The health bonuses are worth having, since anything you do to keep your body in the best possible physical condition will prolong your life.

A Practical Summary of the Basic Diet

Let's pause now for a quick and concise review of the important elements of the basic diet. Once you understand the principles you will have no difficulty in arranging your own menus, whether you are eating at home or dining out.

1. The less you eat the better.
2. The less you weigh the better.
3. Therefore, let the table of optimal weight be your guide to how much you eat.
4. If you are not losing weight—and are now overweight—you are eating too much.
5. The only essential foods appear to be the amino acids of protein, the essential fatty acids—preferably polyunsaturated—and vitamins, minerals, and water.
6. You do not need sugars.
7. The less starch you eat the better.
8. A very small amount of fish, or lean meat, or the whites of hard boiled eggs, or nuts, or skimmed milk or skimmed milk cottage cheese will provide you with the necessary amino acids for good health and long life.
9. If you eat fish daily, you will get a sufficient amount of the essential fatty acids. The Cantor Cocktail (safflower oil linoleic acid) insures an abundance of this polyunsaturated fatty acid.
10. The Longevity Diet, as just outlined, assures an adequate supply of vitamins and minerals. Ocean fish (especially sardines and other herrings) provide vanadium, as well as other minerals and some vitamins.
11. The average fortified skimmed milk used for the Cantor Cocktail has a large amount of vitamin D and A added.
12. Drink three glasses of water between breakfast and lunch and another three glasses between lunch and dinner. These are the essential constituents of the very best basic maintenance diet. Anything you may wish to add to this diet, due to your former habits of sugar and starch, candy and cake eating, only decreases your chance for good health and long life.

The Bonus Supplements You May Use

You may add the bonus supplements of (1) bone meal powder, (2) wheat germ, (3) brewer's yeast. These are natural and good sources of vitamins and minerals and—they are also foods.

If your physician feels that you need a capsule or tablet vitamin-mineral supplement in addition, I have no objection. But it is my opinion that if your water is well-mineralized (hard water), the mineral supplement is not necessary. Besides, the Longevity Diet plus the above listed bonus supplements will certainly give you all that you need of the known essential vitamins and minerals.

Your Health Is in Your Own Hands Through Diet

It is certainly obvious to you by now that how long you will live is largely in your own hands. There is one unknown that we cannot change, and that is the type of tissues you were born with. Some of us are endowed with strong, resistant bodies—so strong and so resistant that we can withstand the slow bullets of diet, tobacco, alcohol and other poisons sometimes well into our sixties and beyond.

Others—and this seems to be most of us—are born with average tissues, and the slow bullets will surely find their mark in our vital organs before we get into or beyond our middle years.

This means that what you do with your new Longevity Key—the magical key of moderation and diet—will determine whether or not *you* become a premature coronary death statistic.

More Tips on Better Living

Since you have stayed with me to this point, I assume that you are serious about better health and longer life. Alright, then, let's once again see what we can do to make life more interesting and more fun.

If you were lucky enough to be born with a cheerful disposition, life is already fun for you. You probably don't have much money (few millionaires have a cheerful disposition), but you are having a barrel of fun. Wonderful!

For those of us who were not so lucky, let's see what we can do to change our ways of thinking. Disposition, after all, is just our way of looking at things, our attitudes toward life. I have a little notebook in which I collect the ideas that are so true that we call them clichés and shrug them off. But they are worth taking seriously. Let's look at a few:

Never look back.

Lot's wife looked back and turned into a pillar of salt. By this I mean that you must not spend your time regretting the errors of the past. It will only make you unhappy, sour your disposition, and spoil your ability to enjoy the present.

Keep smiling.

When you smile you feel better. I keep telling you to try it, and I hope you are making it a habit. It will help change your disposition.

Look for the silver lining.

Now there's a cliché, but it's worth repeating and acting on this advice. Nothing is *all* good or *all* bad, so look for that little bit of good in the bad, and try to turn it to your advantage.

When Fate hands you a lemon, make lemonade.

That's Dale Carnegie's advice, and it is very good. It fits in with the silver lining idea. But remember that it is up to *you* to make the lemonade. Don't just sit around and mope over your bad luck. Do something about it. Make lemonade.

Don't cry before you are hurt.

Most of us spend our days worrying about things that never happen. You will have time enough to cry when they do happen— and *if* they do happen. For the time being—and for always—learn to live one day at a time, forgetting the past and planning (but without fear) for the future. Jesus said it well when he told us:

Sufficient unto the day are the cares thereof.

One day at a time is the best way to live. Get some fun out of today—RIGHT NOW. This is the only day you will ever have, for all you know. For that matter, life is made up only of todays for all of us. Yesterday is gone, tomorrow may never come, and we are left with our todays. Learn to enjoy each and every one of them to the full.

Get the fun habit.

And finally, I will leave you with the important realization that YOU ARE STILL ALIVE. *Survival is all that counts*—at all costs.

Stay alive, and you will have many more opportunities to get rich, become famous, and best of all—TO HAVE FUN.

And NOW, in summary...

1. You and I have reviewed your progress to this point. You know now that your life depends upon how you use the information I have given you in each of these consultations.
2. It will do you good to make a practice of going back over at least one consultation each day.
3. You have learned that there is no single diet pattern and no single food essential for life. You can arrange your own menus once you understand the principles of the Longevity Diet.
4. Stay away from fad diets and fad foods—no matter who recommends them.
5. You have learned the proper food combinations, and the right food sources for the basic essential elements.
6. You have seen, by actual case examples, how too much of a good thing can be deadly. Moderation—even of the essential foods—is your keynote.
7. The less you eat (within reason) the longer you will live. Your guide must be your weight, and the optimal weight chart will give you your proper level.
8. I have given you the facts on calorie calculations.
9. Now you know the precise answers to the questions: How many calories? How much fat? How much protein? How much vitamins and minerals?
10. You know where to get the best quality protein, fats, vitamins and minerals.
11. We have talked still more about the modified vegetarian diet.
12. You have learned about the very special bonus food supplements.
13. You know the twelve vital principles of the basic diet.
14. I have given you more tips on happier living.

CHAPTER 12

YOUR PRESCRIPTION
FOR THE
LONGEVITY DIET

We are rapidly approaching the end of this series of consultations on the First Key to Longevity, the Nutrition Key.

I hope that you are applying everything you have learned, and that you refer back to one of the previous chapter consultations each day, even as you move forward with me in the present one. It is essential to refresh your memory and strengthen your new patterns of eating and thinking by this continuous practice and study. Once the principles become ingrained in your thinking, the new patterns of eating will become second nature, easier and easier to follow. And then you will begin to truly enjoy your food, your new figure, your renewed vitality and youth. You will wonder how you ever ate those enormous, heavy, heart-burdening meals. The killer fats will almost turn your stomach, and when you see others eating as you used to eat, you will think of pigs at a trough, and it will disgust you.

Emphasizing Some Basic Principles You Have
Learned So Far in This Book

I want to leave diet for a brief moment to emphasize a few of the other points in the atherosclerosis puzzle, important points from the SUICIDE CHART. I do this since it is very necessary that you

156

do not fire any of the slow bullets at your vital organs, for the slow bullets of tobacco, stress and insufficient exercise are just as deadly as those of hard fats and cholesterol. Please go back now to our eighth chapter consultation and review the SUDDEN DEATH CHART.

I hope that you have stopped smoking. I hope that you have gone back to dancing—not only when you are out on the town, but even at home. You can dance by yourself, without a partner, whenever the spirit moves you. Humming or singing will do if you do not have a radio, television, or record player for accompaniment. And don't neglect your daily walks, an excellent form of exercise. Any form of noncompetitive exercise will help you limber up your muscles, strengthen your heart and lower your blood cholesterol. I will tell you more about exercise in another consultation chapter. You will find a practical summary of the basic diet in the previous chapter. Review those principles until you know them by heart, for it is *your* heart that is at stake.

In essence: The less you weigh the better, and the table of optimal weights in this book should be your guide.

- No more sugar—certainly not the sugar bowl or candy type.
- Eat fish each day, especially ocean fish.
- Drink your Cantor Cocktail before each meal.
- Drink six glasses of water each day.
- Eliminate the hard meat fats and the dangerous dairy foods you now know about.

Coronary Attack Is a "C" Disease

Here is an interesting observation that will help you remember the principles of the Longevity Diet and the Longevity pattern of living. Coronary artery disease is caused by various factors, each beginning with the letter "C":

Calories	Cookies
Carbohydrates	Cholesterol
Cake	Cigarettes
Candy	

Add this little memory jogger to the one on the SEDENTARY Disease (page 133), and you will have two very good aids to remembering the problem areas.

How Mary Learned the Hard Way to Avoid Being a "C" Casualty

Mary, a patient of mine, comes to mind at this point since she is another C—a Contrary person. She did exactly the opposite of everything she was told to do, a real rebel against life who almost paid the supreme price for her rebellion.

She was only 51 years old, but she looked many years older. She was 40 pounds overweight, and had an elevated blood pressure to match. Her diet and her constant rebellion caused her stomach to speak the organ language of peptic ulcer, with constant heartburn and distress in the "pit of the stomach." The X ray confirmed this diagnosis.

She worked for a magazine and had considerable seniority, but she was always worried because, "So many magazines are folding these days." The combination of stress, poor eating habits, wrong foods, and fear was rapidly terminating her life.

But in spite of this, she did not follow instructions, and rapidly became worse. When I asked her what she was really eating, she told me that one of her neighbors had cured her husband's ulcer by the half milk, half cream diet. This, of course, is a coronary killer, and I told her so. I also advised her that if she kept on this way, surgical removal of the stomach would probably be her only way out.

Regrettably, her rebellion went all the way, and surgery was necessary to stop the hemorrhaging from the ulcer. It was only then —almost too late—that she learned her lesson.

Now, on the proper Longevity Diet, and after training in relaxation, she has improved in all ways. Her weight returned to the optimal level, her blood pressure came down, and her personality changed to one of greater calm, better equanimity, more self-control. She had almost been Contrary enough to die—Contrary enough to be a Coronary Casualty. The deadly C of our memory jogger at work firing the Cholesterol bullets.

Two Basic Diet Questions and Their Answers

Now that you have considered the facts in the previous consultation chapter on the Basic Diet, you must ask yourself two basic questions:

1. *How much* should I eat?
2. *What* should I eat?

The simple answers to these questions form the basis for the Longevity Diet:

1. The less you eat, the better.
2. Stay as close as possible to the basic diet requirements, being particularly careful of the ratio of saturated to unsaturated fats.

In this consultation we will see how these two guiding principles will lead us into a new, healthier world of successful long life.

A One-Day Longevity Plan

Let me tell you my own daily diet to give you an idea of how the Longevity Diet works in actual practice. For breakfast I have orange juice or half a grapefruit and the whites of two hard boiled eggs. Sometimes I drink a decaffeinated coffee, taking it black or with skimmed milk, and a noncaloric sweetener.

I also take a specially formulated vitamin-mineral tablet, one that I use for my postoperative patients to help them in healing. Your physician can prescribe this type of supplement for you if he feels it necessary.

Since I drink very little or no milk, outside of the Cantor Cocktail, I also take a calcium gluconate preparation with breakfast (three grams). But remember that neither the vitamin-mineral tablet nor the calcium tablet are absolutely essential. You may prefer to supplement your diet with powdered bone meal, brewer's yeast and wheat germ—the bonus supplements we have already talked about. If you do, you may omit any other supplement, and ignore my own personal approach to supplementation. Either method (or none at all, since your diet will give you all the vitamins and minerals you might reasonably need) will be okay. So much for my breakfast.

I drink three glasses of water (or more) between breakfast and lunch, and another three glasses (or more) between lunch and dinner. I once met a still active, vital, and alert 88-year-old physician who told me that his secret of long life was to drink very large quantities of water and to eat very little solid food. I agree completely.

I prefer to have lunch quietly in my office while listening to music and reading an interesting magazine or book. This meal consists of a tin of sardines in olive oil, one or two tomatoes, and Sanka or Postum. It is my practice to drain off the olive oil and to replace it with safflower oil. On other days I have eight ounces of skimmed milk cottage cheese instead of the sardines. There is no objection to having both if you wish, and if you can afford the calories.

When I decide to have lunch in a restaurant, I go to a seafood restaurant, and order a mixed green salad, followed by broiled striped bass or red snapper. These are my personal preferences, but you may substitute any other ocean fish you prefer. Finish with Sanka or Postum. Occasional coffee is not harmful, but, for heaven's sake, stay well under five cups a day!

My evening meal is the largest of the day for me. It may begin with a slice of melon or fresh fruit cup, although I have been cutting down on calories lately by omitting a first course. I consider a mixed green salad as my first course, in that case. I like a dressing of safflower oil, lemon juice and garlic. You may prefer safflower oil and vinegar. Suit yourself. My main course is fish, but you may prefer a slice of lean beef or a well-cooked lean steak. I like my fish broiled, and add lemon juice. You may prefer to fry your fish in safflower oil, and perhaps cover it with slivers of almonds. This is real gourmet style, and has my approval.

I have reduced the size of my stomach by the half-portion method of eating, and I am usually too full by this time to want any dessert. But if you are still not full, you may have angel food cake, a water sherbert, or a slice of melon or half a grapefruit. You may even have the proverbial nuts to end your meal. And, of course, there is the decaffeinated coffee, Postum or tea. I do not usually have the room or the desire for a liquid at this time. Remember, my stomach is already well filled before I begin any meal, since I have already had my true first course—the Cantor Cocktail.

Overcoming the Problem of Restaurant Eating

What do I order when dining in a restaurant? Breakfast, of course, is no problem. I instruct the waitress to bring me two ten-minute eggs, "cooked really hard." You will have to specify "ten minutes," or they will be less than hard, and the yolk will be a problem for you. I prefer to separate the yolks from the whites, and you had better tell the waitress or they will be served to you mashed together as if they were soft-boiled. I like freshly squeezed orange juice, but if you cannot get it in your neighborhood restaurant, try half a grapefruit or a slice of melon for breakfast, if you want fruit or juice. Please do not overdo the coffee. Try the decaffeinated type, and you will soon learn to like it. Or give Postum a fair trial, and you will find it to be a good hot drink at any meal. Tea is a stimulant, like coffee, so watch the number of cups of tea.

As to lunch, I have already told you my restaurant routine. Every restaurant has one or another type of fish on the menu, but you will do best if you find a restaurant that specializes in seafood. I may even start with a shrimp cocktail in cocktail sauce but only rarely, since my stomach capacity has been reduced by the half-portion approach. Follow this with a salad, with oil and vinegar (usually olive oil is the best you can get in a restaurant, although many New York restaurants now have safflower oil available, on order, for salad or for frying). Then have fish for your main course, followed by your hot drink (if you still have room).

Dinner in a restaurant certainly offers no problems. The variety of choice naturally depends upon the type of restaurant. As at home, I prefer fish as the main course, but I do like chicken livers (broiled) on occasion. With chicken livers I try to get wild rice (splurging on a good grade starch, with the vitamins intact, by contrast with white rice). I try to have vitamin-rich liver once or twice a week. Remember that chicken liver only contains about 4 per cent fat, and 3 per cent of that is unsaturated—a good ratio of saturated to unsaturated fats. And chicken liver has the added advantage of a large amount of thiamine (vitamin B_1).

What about the bread, butter and rolls served in restaurants? If there is a bread and butter charge, send them back and save your money. Don't hesitate to tell the maitre d' or the waiter that you are on a diet. There is no sense paying for something you don't want, and you certainly do not want the bread, rolls, and butter. If you were at home, you would use a soft margarine (at this writing practically all the margarine companies are coming out with soft, highly polyunsaturated margarines). If you eat lobster, it should be served with melted soft margarine for dipping the lobster meat. Okay, gourmet?

Food Fit for a Gourmet

As you can readily see, this is certainly not a starvation diet. On the contrary, it is a gourmet diet. In fact, if the occasion warrants, either at home or in a restaurant, I have no compunction about ordering a small chicken or a Cornish hen stuffed with wild rice as a main course. I usually only eat half the portion served, and if you are with someone who shares your tastes and your desire to stay alive, perhaps you could have the one portion served for two. Obviously, you can do this most easily at home, since the whole family will undoubtedly be on the same half-portion Longevity Diet. All slim, trim, full of energy and overflowing vitality. All on their way to the 100 or more mark.

The Longevity Diet is obviously a liberal one, well balanced and well rounded, and best of all—a gourmet diet.

Incidentally, I have no qualms about an occasional steak when dining out, if the restaurant is not a specialty fish house. The occasional "slip" is acceptable, even if you go all the way and eat it "black and blue" (charred on the outside and rare inside). Naturally you would do best to eat steak at home, if you must, choosing the cheaper but more healthful grades of meat, since they have much less fat. And you will always cut away the gross fat, since you are certainly not looking for trouble. I don't want you to feel imprisoned by your diet. Some of my patients feel that they absolutely "must have a steak," and I say go right ahead whenever the desire is overpowering. Just keep the quantity small, and remember to cut away the excess fat.

I have omitted only one item in my own daily routine—although I have mentioned it in passing many times—and that is the Cantor Cocktail. Later on, in this consultation, we will talk about this vital food combination in detail. I think you will like it.

Case History of John, Who Almost Buried Himself in Ice Cream

I want to digress for a moment to tell you about one of my friends who was another of the fair, fat and forty problems, the kind of problem that usually hits women the hardest. He is a fine artist, and has a charming wife and a fine little daughter. But that is beside the point.

He loves ice cream. He can eat it "by the gallon." I can understand this very well indeed, since I also have loved ice cream just this same way, and found it hard to give up. But in my case the choice was life or death, and I didn't love ice cream that much. I certainly didn't choose to literally bury myself in an ice cream container.

But my artist friend almost did bury himself in ice cream. He had all the evidences of gall bladder disease, even the colic pain of stones passing through the bile ducts. Fortunately he did not obstruct a duct and become jaundiced. He also had a very high blood cholesterol, and since the rest of his diet matched his flair for fat, this was not unexpected. His blood pressure was quite normal, but he was beginning to develop some chest pain on exertion, early evidence of closing coronary arteries. This brought him to his senses only because one of his very close friends had just dropped dead in his early forties.

John decided to take my advice and change his ways. He went all the way, and followed the diet without even an occasional slip. His was a greater will power than any I have seen in a long time, but he said it was easy, since he "loved life," and had a lot of things he still wanted to do.

That is a good way to look at any diet changes you must make. Do you love life? Do you still have unfinished business, a lot of things you would like to do? Do you have children you want to watch grow up? Do you want to see grandchildren, your best evidence of immortality? Once again it becomes obvious that you write your own ticket. You are the captain of your ship, the one who sets the course to long life or early death. You may become your own executioner. Think about that. John eventually required gall bladder surgery to get rid of the cholesterol stones. But he came through the surgery with flying colors, since he was well prepared by his new Longevity Diet and his better exercise and general health habits. He had lost his excess weight, making it much easier for the surgeon at the operating table. He is now a happier, a healthier and a younger man.

Two More Basic Diet Rules

Remember the first two rules a few pages back? (1) The less you eat the better, and, (2) Stay as close as possible to the basic diet requirements, especially the defender fat rule. Now we come to two more rules for your guidance:

3. Omit Carbohydrates (Sugars) in Your Diet Plans. You will notice that in my own diet selections, I have omitted the starches and the sugars wherever possible. Please do the same. For the fourth rule of the Longevity Diet you need only go back to our consultation on the magic minerals. Remember to add ocean fish to your daily menu, especially the readily available and inexpensive sardines and herring. This is the best way to reduce the accumulation of cholesterol in your artery walls, help stop the formation of gallstones, and improve the texture and health of your skin. So, we come to the next rule:

4. Eat fish daily. To this I want to add the reminder to drink at least six glasses of water daily (eight would be even better). Not only will you find the magic minerals in some hard waters, but this natural body fluid will help immeasurably to keep your system clean and free from harmful collections of waste. Both your kidneys and your bowels need water to stay well.

And a further warning on the overflowing coffee or teapot. Keep your coffee or tea down to no more than five cups a day. Both are dangerous for your vital arteries, and both will set your nervous system on edge. An edgy nervous system makes you more responsive to stress, and this, in turn raises your blood cholesterol level.

If you want to sweeten your hot drink use a non-caloric sweetener. If you want to lighten it, use skimmed milk.

The Cantor Cocktail

Now we come to the keystone of the Longevity Diet, the miracle drink you have heard so much about all through these consultations. First I will give you the original formula for the cocktail, and then I will give you the present-day variations—the ones I recommend for you.

The original cocktail was simply one ounce of cold pressed safflower oil (the kind you can get in any health food store), poured on top of one-third glassful of a non-caloric soda (both chilled), taken immediately before each meal. Since I found it difficult to accustom myself to drinking a fatty substance, I looked for a way to make the drink more palatable, tastier. Many of my patients prefer the original formula, and if you do, too, go ahead. It is the basic, essential cocktail, and contains everything you need. A minor variation is to use a blender or any other mixing device, mix the well-chilled safflower oil and soda, and drink rapidly. Taken in this way, the oil cannot be tasted.

But in recent years I have found a variation of my formula that is even more pleasant and more nutritious. This is the modern Cantor Cocktail that I recommend for you.

The New Cantor Cocktail Formula

The new cocktail tastes exactly like a creamy-rich coffee malted milkshake (and you may choose your own flavor from the many types of low caloric sodas now available). You will require a one-ounce measuring glass (a whiskey glass will do, if it is an honest ounce size), and a blender.

The formula consists of two to three ounces of skimmed milk (preferably the vitamin-fortified type now available in all supermarkets and neighborhood grocery stores), one ounce of safflower oil, and three ounces of coffee-flavored low caloric soda. Blend these ingredients in your blender, and take your time to form a frothy, creamy, delicious mixture. Note that all ingredients must be kept well refrigerated.

You may vary the quantity of skimmed milk in any way you like (two to three ounces, or a whole glassful), to suit your own taste and needs. A similar latitude is allowed for the soda, both as to flavor and amount, for variations in taste and texture.

Many of my patients like a one-two-three formula:

Safflower oil	one ounce
Skimmed milk	two ounces
Low calorie soda	three ounces

But there is no rigidity in this formula, and you may adjust it to suit your own tastes and pleasure.

Another good variation is to simply fill the glass almost to the top

with the skimmed milk and then add the ounce of safflower oil and
follow with whatever amount of soda you need to give you the taste
sensation you find most pleasant. In other words, just suit yourself.

After all, the purpose of the milk is to carry the safflower oil in a
natural way. You see, by adding the oil fat to the milk from which
the dairy fat has been removed, you are simply reconstituting the
milk, making homogenized whole milk. All you have done, in effect,
is to replace the killer animal fat by a defender vegetable fat. Simple
enough, once you understand it. And then you add the soda to make
the drink pleasant.

Incidentally, this same formula is most effective in the treatment
of acid indigestion, either of the simple type or that resulting from
peptic ulcer. It is certainly far superior, from a nutritional-athero-
sclerotic viewpoint, to the usual mixture of half cream and half
milk (deadly both for your weight and your blood vessels!).

Another Variation of the Magical Cantor Cocktail

Lately I have added an ounce of wheat germ to my own mixture,
and 2,000 units of Vitamin E. The ounce of wheat germ contains
approximately 32 per cent protein, 44 per cent carbohydrate and 11
per cent wheat germ oil. It also adds many vitamins (and some
minerals):

Thiamin—.50 mg.	50% of minimum daily requirement (MDR)
Riboflavin—.22 mg.	19% of MDR
Niacin—2.0 mg.	20% of MDR
Phosphorus—330 mg.	44% of MDR
Vitamin C—2.8 mg.	9% of MDR
Vitamin D—9.0 Units	2% of MDR
Vitamin E—6.1 mg.	Requirement unknown
Inositol—190 mg.	Unknown
Folic Acid—.09 mg.	Unknown
Vitamin B_6—.31 mg.	Unknown
Vitamin B_{12}—21 mcg.	Unknown
Choline—105 mg.	Unknown
Pantothenic acid—.36 mg.	Unknown
Sodium—1.0 mg.	Unknown
Iron—2.6 mg.	26% of MDR

The vitamin E is in capsule form, from natural sources, as two hundred international unit capsules, and I simply throw in the gelatin

capsules and let the blender do the rest. (This is natural d-alpha-tocopherol and mixed tocopherols, presumably of value in artery and heart health.) Consult your own physician if you want full information on the still experimental vitamin E.

This makes a thicker mixture of the cocktail, and should be given plenty of time in the blender to allow for fuller dispersion and a complete mixture. Then you must drink it without too much delay, to avoid precipitation to the bottom of the glass or the blender. Just shake it up by swishing your glass if this occurs, and drink the whole thing. I like it, and I think you will like it too.

One of My Patient's Variations of the Cantor Cocktail

One of my patients, an inventor and manufacturer, offers an interesting variation of the Cantor Cocktail. In browsing through the "diet section" of a supermarket, he came across a product which was described as a "diet-milk drink." This is a skimmed milk powder in various flavors such as strawberry, chocolate, cherry, and so forth, that is said to be sugar-free, fat-free and contains eleven calories per fluid ounce.

Each package makes a pint of delicious skimmed milk when mixed with cold water, and my patient simply adds two ounces of safflower oil and puts it through his blender. The result is a very tasty Cantor Cocktail for the next two meals. He drinks one instead of lunch and the other just before dinner.

Make Your Own Variations of the Cantor Cocktail

You can do the same with any skimmed milk powder and a diet type of jam. The skimmed milk powder is readily available everywhere in packages which make a quart.* You need only add four glasses of cold water (or less, if you want to make it richer and "creamier"), and four ounces of safflower oil.

Mix in your blender with four to eight teaspoonfuls of diet jam (choose your own flavor). Each teaspoonful of such diet jam usually contains no more than one and a half calories, so add more if your palate demands it, and especially if you are wise enough to drink your cocktail in place of lunch. These variations are not only

---

* Four cocktails, one before each of the next four meals.

fun to make and drink, but are also quite free from any of the psychological problems of the "oily taste" objection. They are truly delicious! See for yourself!

Magical Reducing Actions of the Cantor Cocktail

The Cantor Cocktail serves more than one purpose. In addition to its high concentration of polyunsaturated fatty acid (linoleic acid), it has an almost "magic" reducing action upon the body. When taken before meals, it satisfies the appetite and reduces the desire for a large meal. This feature is of great importance to everyone on the Longevity Diet, but it will be of special interest to those who are overweight. The appetite-satisfying value of the Cantor Cocktail compares very favorably with the appetite-quenching effect of the amphetamine drugs, and it does the job without any dangerous drug effects. The amphetamine preparations—the major ingredient of the many-colored capsules and tablets prescribed by the "diet doctors" —excite the nervous system. They cause great irritability and should be avoided. In fact, it is a good rule to *avoid drugs generally, unless absolutely necessary and prescribed by a physician as a life-saving measure.*

How to Lose Weight Without Drugs

We will have a great deal more to say about this in the next section of this book, the series of consultation chapters on the Second Key to Longevity. But for the moment it is worth noting that although the Longevity Diet is not primarily intended as a reducing diet, it does just that for those of us who are overweight. Obviously it must, since we certainly will never reach our 100 or more years if we carry around excess fat. The burden on the heart is too great.

The Longevity Diet does the weight reducing job in a very natural fashion, and without drugs, because it is the first of the presently popular low sugar and starch diets. It is a half-portion diet, although you can lose weight to a point even if you stuff yourself with the right protein foods. It differs radically from the ordinary low carbohydrate diets in that it keeps you away from the killer fats and from excess alcohol. After all, there is no point in anyone being a skinny drunk with a diseased heart. The Longevity Diet will work through your natural metabolic processes to bring you to the optimal weight level for your age, sex and body structure. You will then remain at that weight level with very little fluctuation from day to day. It is the best way I know to lose weight pleasantly and permanently while eating three adequate meals each day.

Other Bonuses of the Cantor Cocktail

Another important feature of the Cantor Cocktail is that its high fat content acts to slow the emptying of the stomach. This has the advantage of allowing for full digestion in the stomach before food passes on into the small intestine. And, since the food remains in the stomach for a longer time, it takes less to fill and satisfy the appetite. Obviously, the longer food remains in your stomach, the longer you will have that satisfied "full feeling." With the Cantor Cocktail you lose weight, but you never suffer from gnawing "hunger pangs."

Another reason why this cocktail satisfies the appetite is that fat has a so-called high "satiety value." Fat satisfies our appetite center of the brain more than any other food, and the safflower oil of the cocktail does just that.

Still another bonus benefit of the Cocktail is its exceptionally high vitamin E content. The "normal" daily requirement for vitamin E is around 7 mg. and this amount is supplied many times over by the Cocktail. While the full role of this vitamin in human nutrition is not yet completely understood, we know that it plays an important part in oxygenation, and you can be certain that the very large level of vitamin E in your Cantor Cocktail fully protects you.

And finally, the high caloric content of vegetable fat provides an energy source in the special cocktail. Obviously, the Cantor Cocktail before meals has many advantages and should be the daily keystone of your personal Longevity Diet.

Possible Substitutes for the Cantor Cocktail

A few of my patients find that even with the new formula, they feel a slight nausea—chiefly a psychological reaction to the *thought* of an oily drink. In most such cases, when they fully understand that all they have done is to *make their own homogenized milk* by replacing the killer fat with a safer vegetable fat (safflower oil), the nausea disappears.

However, if the nausea persists, or if there is the least anxiety about the "oily drink" idea, I suggest that the oil content be cut in half. Use only a half ounce of the safflower oil in each cocktail. If this works well, you can then gradually increase the amount until you reach the proper one ounce level. Other—and only very occasional problem patients—speak of bloating and perhaps some diarrhea after being on the cocktail for a few days or weeks.

If this rare problem is yours as well, try cutting the amount in each cocktail to a half ounce of the safflower oil, or eliminate one of the cocktails each day. When your intestinal tract adapts to the new food (more likely when your mind adjusts to the oil drink idea and realizes that it is nothing but reconstituted milk), you will have no further problem. You see, the intestinal tract is the sounding board of the emotions, and reacts quickly when you are disturbed, especially if the distress is more emotional than rational. (See my book, *Ridding Yourself of Psychosomatic Health Wreckers,* if you want to stop such problems for all time).

And finally, for any person who, for one reason or another, does not want to take the cocktail (or who finds it inconvenient when away from home), my advice is to use large quantities of safflower oil with vinegar or lemon juice (and garlic, if you like), as a salad dressing. In this way it is possible to take at least two ounces of the defender fats, one ounce with each salad. Naturally, you will get the greatest benefit if you will learn to enjoy your Cantor Cocktail in modern dress—exactly as described—each day from now on.

Believe me, it is a delicious drink, and you can experiment and adjust the texture and flavor to suit yourself. Have fun on your way to longer life and better health.

The Lucky Seven Commandments of Longer Life

If we now put together all the vital principles of the First Key to Longevity—the Key of Nutrition—we have the "Lucky Seven Commandments of the Cantor Longevity Diet."

1. The less you eat, the better.

2. The less you weigh, the better (your body will find the "right" weight level, if you will just give it a chance.

3. Forget Carbohydrates.

4. Eat fish daily.

5. Drink at least six glasses of water daily.

6. Drink the Cantor Cocktail before each meal.

7. Obtain the vital amino acids of protein from fish, lean meat, the white of hard-boiled eggs, and skimmed milk products.

These "Lucky Seven" are really the only principles you need to know, and a review of the consultation on the Basic Diet will help to strengthen your understanding and recall of these vital ideas. Since the Longevity Diet is a gourmet diet, you will not only live longer by following my teachings, but will have the fun of good eating while doing it.

From now on it is up to you to work out your own menus, using these Lucky Seven principles. The possible variety is limited only by your own ingenuity.

To help you in the selection of the Longevity meals, I will now give you some food lists and tables. These are simply general guides to help you apply the Lucky Seven principles. But always remember that your truly basic guides are: eat as little as possible, let your weight be your guide (rather than calorie counting), and maintain a high ratio of the defender polyunsaturated fats as compared with the killer saturated fats (while keeping the total amount of fats of all kinds to a low level).

How the Lucky Seven Commandments Helped
One Family Avoid Slow Suicide

This family was well on its way to slow bullet suicide when I first met the 41-year old mother. She was complaining of fatigue, and I did not think this unusual when I learned that she had five youngsters ranging from ten to 19, and a large house to look after. Her husband was employed in a supermarket, and they did not lack for food. As a matter of fact, they all ate too much of the high starch and high sugar foods, following the pattern set down by her own mother.

"Bread is the staff of life, I always say," is exactly what she believed and put into action.

I pointed out that bread used to be the staff of life in the days when it was baked at home, for then it contained all the vitamins and other nutrients of the whole grain, and none of the chemical additives of today's bread. I suggested that it was now a very weak staff, and one that might even be dangerous.

This patient had other complaints, including headache and backache, severe constipation, and some blood in her bowel movements. She had a small, nonmalignant growth in her rectum, and I promptly removed it in my office. That stopped the bleeding. I then did a blood study, and found that she had a very high cholesterol level, and was also on the verge of a diabetic level of blood sugar. Her blood pressure was normal.

Every member of this family was overweight—as you would expect from their high sugar and high starch diet. The transformation when they all went on the Longevity Diet was wonderful to behold.

She grasped the Lucky Seven Commandments at once, and had the good sense to give up her food suicide habits. Weight came down to normal, the whole family had more energy than ever, and my patient looked younger and prettier than her chronological age called for. That is one of the major rewards of the Longevity Diet— it rolls back the years and turns back the biological clock. And now for the promised food lists, so you can start to do the same for yourself, creating your own gourmet Longevity meals as follows.

Foods You Should Eat Daily

1. Fish, especially sardines, herring and ocean fish.
2. Safflower (or corn oil)—three ounces daily.
3. A large mixed green vegetable salad with tomatoes, once or twice a day, with safflower oil and vinegar dressing. Add garlic or other seasoning to taste.
4. Skim milk cottage cheese, skim milk, or buttermilk (for calcium, phosphorus, potassium, and protein).
5. Six to eight glasses of water daily.
6. Those who do not enjoy fish may substitute lean beef, foul, veal, lamb, liver, nuts. The best protein course is ocean fish. After fish, we would list the whites of hard-boiled eggs, followed by skim milk, cottage cheese and buttermilk. Of animal protein sources, the next best is fowl. Liver is next. Veal follows. Nuts are an excellent protein source, and I would recommend almonds, roasted cashews, pecans, walnuts and roasted peanuts. These nuts provide a valu-

able protein combined with a high unsaturated fat, low saturated fat content.

Recommended Edible Oils

1. Safflower oil (88 to 90 per cent unsaturated fatty acid content—chiefly polyunsaturated).
2. Corn oil (85 per cent unsaturated fatty acid content—largely polyunsaturated and monounsaturated).
3. Sunflower oil (90 per cent unsaturated fatty acid content).
4. Soy bean oil (80 per cent unsaturated fatty acid content—largely polyunsaturated and monounsaturated).
5. Olive oil (88 per cent unsaturated fatty acid content—chiefly monounsaturated). Safflower oil contains a very high percentage of the "essential" fatty acid, lineolic acid. However, if it is not available, corn oil may be used with very good effect.

The Preferred Foods

1. All fish and sea foods. (If served fried, use safflower or corn oil).
2. The whites of hard-boiled eggs.
3. Skim milk cottage cheese. (This food may be made more palatable for some people by adding additional skim milk, chopped vegetables, fruits, or nuts or spices to taste.)
4. Skim milk.
5. Buttermilk (made from skim milk).
6. Vegetable oils, especially safflower and corn oil.
7. All fruits.
8. All vegetables.
9. Poultry, preferred in the following order:
   chicken—white meat
   chicken—dark meat
   pheasant
   quail
   squab
   turkey
   duck (cook out all the fat)
10. Meats, preferred in the following order:
   chicken liver
   beef liver
   calf liver
   veal
   leg of lamb
   lean beef
11. Nuts:
   pecans

walnuts
almonds
cashews
peanuts

Acceptable Only For Those Not Overweight (But Not Preferred)

1. Whole grain bread.
2. Angel food cake.
3. Oatmeal.
4. Branflakes.
5. Farina.
6. Shredded Wheat.

Food Supplements

1. Wheat germ.
2. Brewer's yeast.
3. Bonemeal powder.

Forbidden Foods

1. All baked goods other than angel food cake.
2. All breads other than whole grain breads.
3. Macaroni, spaghetti, noodles (especially egg noodles).
4. All hard cheese.
5. All processed cheese, hard or soft.
6. Butter.
7. Lard.
8. All margarine *except nonhydrogenated margarines.*
9. Whole milk.
10. Milk sherbet.
11. Mayonnaise.
12. Coconut oil.
13. All hydrogenated shortenings.
14. All salad dressings other than those prepared with safflower oil or corn oil.
15. All gravies, flour and meals with the exception of oatmeal.
16. All pork and pork products.
17. All other meats not listed as preferred.
18. All sugars and sweets, including candy, chocolate syrup, jams, jellies, and marmalades. (A small amount of pure honey may be permitted if you are not overweight).
19. All prepared meats, smoked meats, delicatessen.

Alcohol

The rule is the less the better. None at all is best, but if your habit is an occasional drink, continue it, unless you are overweight.

Alcohol has more calories than most people imagine. There are 100 calories in 6 ounces of beer, 72 calories in one wine glass of dry red wine, 158 calories in a wine glass of muscatel or port, and 85 calories in dry champagne.

One and one-half ounces of whisky ranges from 105-115 calories.

The popular Martini tops the list with 166 calories in a three ounce glass, while a Manhattan offers 151 calories per three ounces.

Summing It All Up

You now know the best principles of the Longevity Diet, how they were derived, and their relationship to improved health and longer life. You also know how I have applied them in my own life, and what they have done for me. It only remains for you to determine what this diet can do for you. Now that you know the principles involved, you can make your dietary selections intelligently and not blindly. You now know why a particular food should be eaten, and why another one should be avoided.

When these principles become second nature to you, the life of a gourmet will be yours; you will have increasing vitality and energy, improved mental attitude, a slim-trim figure, and a long life.

Lift your Cantor Cocktail high. Here's to the new person with a long bright future—YOU!

More Tips for Better Living

Your Longevity Diet will give you greater energy and more vitality than you have experienced in years. What will you do with the new energy?

I would suggest that you keep busy, keep active, keep working. Stay on the job, and if you have no regular work, see what you can do with a new hobby.

Try painting. Grandma Moses did it, and it kept her happy and young well into her nineties. It also made a great deal of money. Or *try writing.* You may find you have a talent for it. Start with your own life story, from childhood on to the present moment. This is great therapy, one that will help you get rid of much of the emotional turmoil of your past, just as if you were lying on the psychoanalyst's couch pouring out all your past troubles to him. Pour them out on paper, and you will be astonished at how much better you feel after each writing session.

When you finish this writing therapy you may find yourself with

a best seller on your hands. Frank and personal writing has a large
market these days.

Another good way to use your new energy is to join in those
civic activities or church activities you probably have been neglect-
ing. *Help others* (to help yourself). When you give of yourself, this
is true giving. And it will make you happier and healthier at the
same time. It will make you a better person. It will keep you young
when you start forgetting about your own aches and pains and worries, and start thinking about others. Most of all, *practice smiling
and enthusiasm.* You will find that it is contagious. A smile, a laugh,
a hug and a kiss—these are the best medicines. Use them regularly.

And NOW, in summary . . .

1. We have reviewed your progress to this point, and have
   given you more tips for better health.
2. We have reviewed the basic principles of the Basic Diet.
3. You have learned why I call Coronary artery problems a
   "C" disease, and how to overcome all of the "C" factors.
4. My own One Day Longevity Plan is now yours.
5. Now you know how to eat at home and in restaurants—
   foods for fun and long life.
6. You have been instructed in the four Basic Rules.
7. The mysteries of the Cantor Cocktail and its many bonuses are now revealed.
8. The many variations of the Cantor Cocktail are fun to
   mix and fun to drink.
9. My own Cantor Cocktail formula is revealed.
10. You can now lose weight without drugs, while shedding
    both pounds and years. You can turn back the biological
    clock.
11. The Lucky Seven Commandments, your basic Longevity
    Diet principles, are listed for you.
12. You have learned the lessons of interesting problem cases.
13. More tips for better living will help you get more fun out
    of your new vitality and your new energy.

YOUR SECOND KEY
TO LONGEVITY

CHAPTER 13

EXERCISE FOR HEALTH AND LONGEVITY CAN BE FUN

When you have put the vital rules of the previous consultations into daily action, you will have left the food-suicide class and "joined" the International Anti-Coronary Club. Even though you are only an unofficial member at this point, you are most welcome. We expect to have you with us for at least 100 years. If you want to join officially, drop me a note at the UNITROL Teaching Institute.* I will be glad to hear from you, and to learn of your progress toward better health, a new slim and trim figure, and longer life. We will set up the club rules and regulations, and arrange for regular publications on new developments in longevity to reach you without delay. Let's do it together for the good of all who want to leave the food-suicide group, all who want to live a longer and a happier life.

The Truth About Exercise

You will always hear many confusing statements on the importance of exercise and its dangers. Exercise is both important and dangerous, and moderation remains our keynote here as in all else.

---

* 147-41 Sanford Ave., Flushing, 11355, N.Y.

I have told you something about exercise during our previous consultations, and this is a good time to review the facts.

You will remember that exercise can lower blood cholesterol. I told you about the study of Irish brothers, some living in Ireland and some in Boston, and how the Irish group had a lower blood cholesterol than the Boston group despite their high fat diet. The answer was simply that the group of brothers in Ireland were much more active in their daily lives than their Boston brothers. The activity and exercise of their daily lives brought down their blood cholesterol level. So exercise is important in preventing coronary artery disease and sudden death.

The Value of Calisthenics

I do not approve of violent calisthenics, rigorous exercise, or competitive games—unless you are a trained athlete. The kind of exercise I am talking about—the kind that will bring down your blood cholesterol—is simply the kind that any busy man or woman who works with their hands would be doing. This kind of normal activity improves your circulation, helps maintain proper muscle tone, and keeps your joints and muscles limber.

But if you are unaccustomed to strenuous exercise, strenuous work, or competitive sports, you must begin slowly and gradually, going a little further each day. The simplest and best form of exercise is walking, and I want to talk about that for a few moments.

The Oldest Form of Exercise Is Good for All of Us

Walking comes naturally to all of us. It is truly the oldest and the most natural form of exercise for all ages. A simple walk each morning—about one hour—will give you all the exercise you need, and is an excellent way to start your day. If necessary, get up an hour earlier and take your morning walk. This is the old-fashioned constitutional, and it is great exercise as well as good fun.

During your walk, look around you and really *try to see*. Listen to the sounds of the country or the city. *Try to hear*. Most of us look but do not see, listen but do not hear. We are not really living until we learn to see, to hear, to feel, to taste, to smell. These are the ways your body and mind contact the reality of life. Use them and you will be living more fully than you ever have before. Train yourself to see and hear during your morning walks. It's great and you'll love the new experience. Not only that, you will come back refreshed, revitalized, full of new energy and a new appreciation of life. What a wonderful way to start the day!

A Magical Secret to Use when Walking

And now for a little secret you can use to grow younger while walking. Simply talk to your subconscious mind with each step. In time with your body rhythm, repeat to yourself over and over: *"Younger and Younger, Younger and Younger, Younger and Younger. . . ."*

This will act as a command to your subconscious mind. Since this control center of your nervous system takes everything literally, it will accept this command and put all your body forces into action to make you younger. It will mobilize your endocrine glands and all your vital tissues to bring your command into being.

Do this with each step, each day, throughout the entire walk, and you will find your steps becoming more vigorous, with a new and younger bounce, a new and younger rhythm, a new and younger joy in living.

If you want to learn more about how this works, I would suggest that you read my book, *UNITROL: The Healing Magic of The Mind.* For the moment, however, all you have to do is to put this "magic" to work, and see for yourself.

Walking Strengthens Your Heart

Exercise like walking not only lowers your blood cholesterol, but it also strengthens your heart muscle. Don't walk or do any other form of exercise beyond the limits of your normal endurance. As you become stronger, as your heart adjusts to the gradually longer and longer walks, this vital muscle strengthens. At the same time your breathing improves, strengthening the muscles of respiration and your lungs.

The fresh morning air, relatively free from automobile exhaust and other fumes, brings healing oxygen into your blood stream to help nourish your revitalized muscles and all other tissues. Sun or rain, just like the mailman on his appointed rounds, take your youth-building morning walk.

The Bicycle

Did you ride a "bike" when you were a kid? This is a good time to begin again and to recapture the spirit of youth while getting that vital exercise.

The famous heart specialist, Dr. Paul Dudley White, recommends bicycle riding as one of the best forms of exercise. But be sure to do it gradually—a little more each day—so you do not put too much strain on your body the first time out. If you approach this form of exercise in a slow and gradual way, you will soon be riding many miles each day, rebuilding your energies, your muscles and your heart and lungs. But take it easy at first, and only go a little further each day, if you want the best possible degree of benefit from this fine exercise.

You Can Dance Your Way to Youth

During one of our previous consultations I recommended dancing to you. I even told you about dancing in bed by contracting and relaxing the muscles of your arms and legs in time to the music of radio, record player or television. This is an excellent way to combine relaxation with safe and pleasant muscle action. You do not move the joints when you do this rhythmic muscle movement. This is fun, and I guarantee you that you will enjoy "dancing in bed!" At the same time, it tires your muscles just enough to help you slip off into restful sleep.

As you practice this restful and fun-way of exercising, you will be surprised to see how your control of individual muscle groups improves. You will be able to contract and relax any muscle you choose, just by thinking about it. After all, your mind controls your muscles, so this should be no surprise to you.

You Can Slim Down with Bed Exercises

What may be a surprise to you is the fact that this very simple and pleasant way of exercising in bed will trim inches off your measurements. At the same time that you are losing pounds, you will be losing inches from your waistline if you learn to contract and relax your abdominal muscles. This is quite easy with practice. We can say the same for the thighs, the calves, and so on. All you have to do is to "point your mind" at the muscles you want to move, and they will move. Each time they do they will become tighter, stronger and healthier. As their tone improves, your measurements shrink. You will have learned another way to a slim and trim body to supplement the effect of your Longevity Diet.

Benefits of Eccentric Dancing

Another fun-way to exercise is eccentric dancing. Do this in the privacy of your bedroom. Strip down to your underwear, or put on some comfortable and nonrestricting clothing, and turn on your radio or record player. Now dance around the room any way you please, in time to the music. The whole family can do this together, if they wish, or you can do it alone. It's good fun to just dance around the room, making up your own steps, moving in time to the music. This is really the essence of modern dancing.

You can bring your whole body into action, or you might just feel like moving your arms and hands or your head. Perhaps you will simply swing gracefully from the hips while staying in one place. Be as casual and relaxed and eccentric as you wish. Make it fun, and it will do you the most good.

Add an hour of eccentric dancing to your daily activity schedule, just before going to bed. Follow this with the muscle dance in bed —perhaps while watching television—and then slip off into your restful, revitalizing sleep of youth.

Golf Can Be Fun, but—

Golf can be fun, and it can be useful to help you build your heart and body—but it can also be deadly. I remember one of my good friends, only 51 years old, who took his golf too seriously. He was always competing against himself, trying to improve his swing, trying to beat his score the last time around.

He had high blood pressure, and he was much too heavy from rich food and too much liquor. So I warned him against golf. But it was useful for business contacts, and he said, "I enjoy the game, so don't worry." One day he suffered a stroke and died at the ninth hole. It was his last time around.

Now that doesn't mean that you can't play golf. What it does mean is that you must not take it too seriously. Don't keep score necessarily. Play for the exercise. Play for the fun. And if it isn't fun—quit! The game, then, is not for you. Give it up and stay alive longer.

Golf and Substitute Aggression

Golf can be used for a form of therapy I call Substitute Aggression. Think of the golf ball as your wife, your boss, your husband, that vicious neighbor, that cut-throat business competitor—anyone who may be "in your hair" at the time—and whack the devil out of the ball. "Cuss" aloud if you're alone, or under your breath if you are playing with others.

You will be surprised at how much better you will feel after each solid whack at the little ball—that substitute for the person you really want to take a poke at. This is a safe way to let off dangerous steam that might otherwise play havoc with your own body. It may save you from a coronary attack, a stroke, or some other form of organ language warning. In this way you will be combining the benefits of exercise with the release of stress—and both factors will help lower your blood cholesterol.

Riding the Imaginary Bicycle

You do not even need a bicycle to enjoy the leg motions of riding. All you need to do is to lie on your back and pedal in the air, slowly or rapidly, to ride your imaginary bicycle. This will give you the benefit of exercise. You should do it gradually, only to the point of tiring your legs. Little by little, day by day, you will be able to pedal your imaginary bicycle further and further.

Naturally, this is not exactly equivalent to riding the real thing, since you lose the benefit of being outdoors, the fresh air, and the sense of adventure, as well as the exercise of other parts of your body while pedaling a bicycle. But it will do as a starter, and even as a permanent substitute if you do not know how to ride a bicycle, or prefer not to. The important thing is the exercise, since your objective is not to build strong muscles (although you will do this as you go along), but to strengthen your heart and arteries while lowering your blood cholesterol level.

The Case of Harry, Who Believed in Taking Chances with His Health

This patient should have been called Hairbreadth-Harry, because he really believed in taking chances. Seventy pounds overweight, 30 years old, unmarried, and with a desk job, he refused to change his diet. Despite my warning him of a very high blood cholesterol level and an equally high blood pressure level, the only part of my advice that he accepted was the recommendation that he exercise.

And here he also showed the Hairbreadth-Harry approach by joining a gymnasium and going at his exercises with a vengeance. This was a suicide approach, and it very nearly cost him his life. He had a small stroke while running against younger men in better condition. This put him literally out of the running for several months, after which he was ready to listen to reason, which simply consisted of the Longevity Diet and exercise in small doses, gradually increasing each day—always without competition.

Harry's blood cholesterol level came down, and so did his elevated blood pressure. He lost his excess weight, and became a more vigorous and more vital person. He even thought of marriage for practically the first time. "I never thought girls would be interested in a fatty," he said.

Jumping Rope

An excellent form of exercise—one that will help take you back to your childhood—is jumping rope. You can use an ordinary piece of clothesline, or you can buy a regular jump rope in a sporting goods store. Better still—and this is the way I prefer to do it—is to simply imagine the rope while you jump. If you imagine the rope you will get the exercise without the frustration of missing a single jump. You can do fancy cross-overs with your arms, and you can jump in any intricate pattern of steps you wish. I find it more fun that way. Try it both for exercise and for fun.

Exercise Without Body Motion

The newest form of exercise is called isometric exercise, which is exercise without moving the joints. I have already told you of one form of exercise in bed in which you simply "point your mind" at your muscles, one after the other, causing them to contract and relax on silent command. If you do not move the joints connected to those muscles, you will be practicing isometric exercise.

If you keep the individual muscle in a state of contraction— tight and bulging—for about six to ten seconds, you will build the size and strength of the muscle. This is a method of muscle strengthening that has been successfully used by Olympic athletes of all countries. It requires no apparatus and is not particularly tiring. I recommend it. If you want to slim your waistline with little effort, all you need do is to tighten your abdominal muscles (stomach muscles), and hold them in the contracted position for at least six seconds. Do this as often as you can, and especially while walking and while sitting. Naturally, you will also do it when you are lying down, before going off to sleep.

Women who do this regularly are soon able to hold in their "stomach" muscles with ease, *and without a girdle.* Men are able to hold the new slim, trim waistline posture without any trouble, and can then draw in their belts a few notches. This is the best way to reduce the waistline while strengthening and exercising essential muscles—even if you do not need to lose weight.

I have learned to control my abdominal muscles to the point that I can roll them up or down at will, very much like a belly dancer. Within a relatively short time, simply by daily practice, you will develop the same control. You will have fun while you are doing it, and you will be getting the essential exercise to help lower your bood cholesterol level. The slimmer waistline will be your added bonus.

Running in Place

If you cannot get out for a walk on any particular day, you might prefer a short run—right in your own room. All you need to do is to get up on your toes and run in place. Do this form of exercise quite gradually, increasing the time each day. You may only wish to run for a minute or two the first day. Certainly you should not run long enough to tire yourself out or to become short of breath. You can run quite slowly or as fast as your general physical condition permits. But always stop short of tiring yourself or becoming winded. Remember—you are doing this to help lower your blood cholesterol, while at the same time increasing your general fitness, your lung capacity and strengthening your heart muscle. You are not doing it as an athlete, and you are not in competition with anyone.

Exercise Versus Coffee Break

In some European countries workers take an exercise rather than a coffee break. This is an excellent idea for several very good reasons. First, as you already know, more than five cups of coffee a day may bring you to, or over, the verge of a coronary artery attack. Second, the exercise will tone up your body and make your blood circulate health-giving oxygen throughout your entire body. Your heart muscle will strengthen, and your lungs will improve their breathing capacity. Your blood cholesterol will move out of the danger zone. Whenever you might ordinarily think of a coffee break, remember that coffee is part of the dangerous C group, the Coronary killer group—and take an exercise break instead. You can practice the muscle contraction type of isometric exercise while sitting at your desk, or you can take a walk. If convenient, you can jump rope with your imaginary rope.

The coffee break can subtly break your health and eventually shorten your life. The exercise break will strengthen your body and prolong your life. Take your choice.

Deskcercise

This is the name I give to the muscle contraction form of exercise—the type I recommended for you while lying in bed—when performed while sitting at your desk. You can do this without calling attention to yourself by simply "pointing your mind" at the muscles of your abdomen, for example, tightening and relaxing, or rolling them like a belly dancer. You can do the same with your leg muscles, one at a time, or both legs at once, alternately tightening and relaxing the selected muscles. Do the same with your arm muscles, your forearm muscles, your shoulder muscles, and so on. It's good fun, does not require you to leave your desk, and you can even do it while working or in conference. Best of all, it helps your heart and arteries.

Avoid the *coffee coronary* by substituting the *exercise energizer*.

A Word of Warning on Exercising

A study of oldsters who have lived beyond the 100 mark shows that a vigorous, active physical life is important. You now know the reasons why. But this does not mean competitive sports or active calisthenics. It does mean a regular pattern of activity—perhaps simply active housework for the ladies and active physical work for the men. If your occupation is sedentary, practice the fun forms of exercising you have just learned. Exercise should always be fun, and it will be if you use eccentric dancing, dancing in bed, and the real or imaginary bicycle riding.

You must always remember that the First Key to Longevity is the magic Key of Nutrition. Exercise is the supplementary Second Key—just like the second key used by the bank attendant when he opens your safety deposit box. *It won't work without the first key.*

And just so that you will not go to excess and become a suicide from exercise, let me tell you that although former college athletes live approximately six months longer than their nonathletic classmates, honor students live a year or two longer than do the athletes! Obviously brains are better than brawn, and you must use your very good brain to follow the teachings of the First Key to Longevity, and practice the Exercise Key method only as a supplement to proper nutrition.

And NOW, in summary . . .

I have enjoyed our visit today, and I hope that you have learned the important facts about the Second Key to Longevity. Let's take a few moments, now, and summarize our consultation.

1. Having learned the vital First Key to Longevity, I now cordially invite you to join with me in the formation of an International Anti-Coronary Club. This will be designed

to bring you the latest information on better health and longer life.

2. I have introduced you to the truth about exercise, and have shown you how it can be both life-saving and dangerous. You must make the choice.

3. Exercise will help you lower your blood cholesterol level and rid your arteries of their cholesterol deposits.

4. Stay away from calisthenics, competitive exercise and other vigorous sports. You are not trying to become an athlete. You just want better health and longer life.

5. Walking is a natural form of exercise, and offers many additional benefits for the lungs and the mind.

6. You have learned the magic secret of combining walking and self-suggestion. It will help make you younger.

7. Bicycle riding is an excellent heart-strengthener, and you can even use an imaginary bicycle.

8. I have taught you the fun way to exercise—eccentric dancing in bed, and even "deskcercise."

9. You know now how to use golf as a heart-saver rather than as a suicide game. It can help you rid yourself of your aggressions.

10. Rope-skipping—even with an imaginary rope—is fun and good for your heart.

11. I have taught you the secret of isometric exercise—but not for muscle building. Use this secret to slim your measurements.

12. This whole consultation chapter has been devoted to the fun way to exercise—one of my best tips for better living and longer life.

YOUR THIRD KEY
TO LONGEVITY

CHAPTER 14

THE MAGICALLY ACTING HORMONES FOR HEALTH, YOUTH, AND LONGEVITY

In this chapter I am going to reveal "real magic"—the "magic" of your own hormones. You will learn what a hormone is, and how some of them work to keep your body young and in good health.

You will learn about the substances that keep a woman young far beyond the ordinary menopause (change of life). You will learn how a woman can prolong her love life—one of the special bonuses of staying young. This is truly a sexual revolution for women, a revolution that permits them to control aging and conception at the same time.

I will also teach you about the lazy thyroid, and how a tiny pill can restore vigor and youth to both men and women. I will show you how this hormone of your thyroid gland, and the estrogenic hormones of women, help to keep your blood cholesterol level down where it belongs. Another bonus of the magic hormones, another key to staying young and healthy.

A Word of Caution

Before going a single step further, I want to caution you against taking any of these powerful hormones without careful supervision

193

by a competent physician. We can talk about them during this consultation, but there is a large gap between talking and using. Do not try to cross that gap by yourself. Do it hand in hand with your doctor.

What Is a Hormone?

Perhaps you are already familiar with the endocrine glands. For a brief review, I want to refresh your memory. The endocrine glands we want to talk about today are the ovaries of women, men's testicles, and the thyroid gland. An endocrine gland you are undoubtedly familiar with is the pancreas, for this is the gland that pours insulin into our bodies to help us burn up sugar foods. If we do not produce enough insulin we are diabetic, and need to take this hormone by injection, or by mouth.

The endocrine glands also include the four parathyroids, the master pituitary gland at the base of the brain, the two adrenals perched on top of our kidneys, and the thymus and the pineal gland (both still little understood). The pancreas is the largest, and all the others are quite small, yet these bundles of tissue literally make us what we are.

If they function correctly, we are healthy, alert and vigorous. If they fail, we become sick, old, and often die. These are the glands that secrete the magical hormones—chemical substances that pour directly from the glands into the blood stream. And it is these hormones that control all the other tissues of our body.

Hormones' Influence on the Body

These powerful chemicals were practically unknown a hundred years ago. Now we understand that they are the chemical keys to health and long life. When we learn enough about them, how to prepare them in the laboratory, how to put them in potent pill or injection form, how to use them to bolster failing natural hormone production by the endocrine glands, we will be well on our way to chemical control of every body function and the length of our lives. We can already do this with the ovarian hormones—and we are learning more about how to use them to prolong youth with each passing day. And we can do this with the thyroid hormone, as I will tell you later on when we talk about the lazy thyroid. Many physicians are now well acquainted with these powerful hormones, and can advise you in their use.

Hormones Are Life-Force Regulators

These hormones are truly life regulators, controlling all body systems, all organ functions, all tissue and cellular health. They tell the tissues whether to grow tall and strong, or short and stunted. They tell the nervous system whether to be alert and perhaps even brilliant to a genius level, or dull, stupid, or even imbecilic. They control the beating of the heart and the functions of the kidneys, liver, bones, muscles, and joints. They control the intestinal tract and the blood stream defense system. In brief, they control everything on the basic life-force level.

For the moment we are especially concerned with the hormones of sex—and most especially the female sex hormones, estrogen and progesterone. We know now that the female sex hormones can be used to postpone the menopause indefinitely, while controlling conception at the same time. And we know that this can be done safely.

We also know that the male sex hormones, testosterone or its synthetic analogs, can control the symptoms of the male menopause for men beyond their fifties. New vigor and vitality, prevention of depressions and diminished work capacity, are some of the benefits of male sex hormone treatment. There are even hormone synthetics to prevent enlargement of the prostate gland. We will have much more to say about both female and male sex hormone therapy, since this is a major Key to Longevity.

The Sexual Revolution

We are now in the early stages of a true sexual revolution. There are women now taking "the pill" who will retain their full femininity as long as they live. They will be *women* in the best sense of the word—not only physically, but also emotionally, forever. This is a form of youth prolongation that is now available to practically all women.

They will be permanently young! Doctors now are beginning to think of the menopause as they do of diabetes—as a deficiency disease *rather than as a natural life process*. Of course, this is not entirely comparable, since it is indeed the natural course of events for women to stop menstruating and to stop bearing children when they reach a certain age. But it is true that the *change of life is due to a deficiency in the sex hormones,* just as insulin is lacking in the diabetic patient. And it is true that the female sex hormones will "cure" the deficiency and keep women young, supple and free from the change of life symptoms indefinitely.

How to Become a "Permanently" Young Woman

How would you like to remain constantly young? It may be possible for you. Let's define exactly what this will mean to you. Your skin will remain firm, supple, softly textured and smooth. Your bones will not lose their calcium and become brittle. They will remain strong and young, holding your body erect and tall. Your muscles will keep their youthful strength and resiliency. You will not develop the "dowager's hump," and you will keep your youthful grace and fluidity of motion.

You will not have the hot flushes, the irritability and depression, the anxiety and crying spells, the many other symptoms that are often associated with menopause.

Heart Insurance with Hormones

The female sex hormones give the fertile female—before the menopause—a special protection against coronary artery disease. We have already spoken of this in an earlier consultation chapter. When you take these same hormones during the menopause—and indefinitely postpone the change of life—you will be giving yourself continuing protection against coronary artery disease. This is a form of heart insurance that is available to men, also, but at a price. They become feminized—a rather high price, but one that some men will gladly pay rather than be prone to repeated heart attacks.

Let me tell you about one such man in the following case.

Case History of a Male Taking Female Hormones for Heart Disease

This male patient was 54 years old when he had his first coronary closure. He persisted in the suicide pattern of the C disease (see page 157), and refused to give up smoking, fatty foods, sweet desserts and his 12 cups of coffee each day. His second coronary closure nearly ended his life two years later. It was then that I told him about the female sex hormone insurance, and the protection that it might give him. He decided that he no longer wanted to be a willful suicide, and started on the complete Longevity Program. He also chose to take the female sex hormones, despite the full understanding that they might cause femininizing changes in him.

His breasts enlarged and his beard became somewhat sparse. His hips enlarged. He lost his sexual potency to a large degree. Nevertheless, he was willing to pay the price in order to stay alive. It is safe to predict that the time will come when a non-feminizing synthetic hormone will come out of the laboratory to help protect the suffering male against fat deposits in his coronary arteries.

Is Aging a "Deficiency" Disease?

It may well be that many of the changes of aging should be considered evidences of a deficiency disease. Certainly this is the thinking of some doctors who treat the menopause as a deficiency disease. To prevent the aging changes that go with the change of life we need only prescribe the missing hormones, thus correcting the deficiency.

This does not mean that the female sex hormones need be prescribed routinely for all women during the menopause. Some have a good hormone balance during that time, and they do not age rapidly (perhaps as many as 15 per cent of all women are this lucky). But the careful use of the magic hormones for all other women will prevent the menopause and all its suffering, all its unpleasant emotional and physical changes.

How Hormones Proved to Be the Key in Curing a General Run-Down Condition

I remember this lovely woman of 45 who was referred to me for symptoms of poor intestinal track function. She had been treated for a chronic stomach ulcer, based on her symptoms of heartburn, poor digestion, and questionable X ray studies that were "not quite definite." She went to many doctors seeking relief. Her problem turned out to be one of the symptoms of the change of life. The magic female sex hormones relieved her completely, unmasking the real culprit.

The moral of our story is that many women complain of symptoms relating to any and all parts of the body during the menopause, and the physician must not be caught in the trap of treating symptoms rather than the disease. These women may go from one specialist to another, looking for the answer to general weakness, headaches, backaches, skin, bone or joint distress, and almost anything else you can think of. They naturally deserve a very complete study before writing off these symptoms as evidence of the menopausal deficiency. But once the studies are completed and once the decision is made that there is no serious disease in any part of the body, the magical hormones should be used. They may provide the answer for restoration of health for a longer life.

Body Changes and the Therapeutic Test

If a woman in the menopausal age group shows any of the following body changes, she is a candidate for a trial run of the female hormones:

Dowager's hump.
Coronary changes on electrocardiogram studies (or symptoms of this problem).
Shrinking physical size (due to loss of bone calcium and other spine changes).
Brittle bones.
Skin dryness and sagging.

Muscle weakness.

Flabby breasts.

Vaginal irritation, inflammation and dryness.

Scrawney neck.

Gaunt extremities.

Perhaps stiff joints and other evidences of aging.

Undiagnosed general physical and mental disturbances.

What do we mean by the therapeutic test? Simply that the physician, after a careful study that shows no specific disease, tries the estrogenic hormones to see whether or not they will relieve the patient's symptoms. Since the magical hormones are relatively harmless when carefully prescribed and supervised by the doctor, they should be tried in every such problem female. The results may well exceed your expectations.

I am trying to show you how to live a happier and healthier, as well as a longer life, and the magical hormones will certainly slow down the aging rate for you. They will certainly correct the physical and mental changes of the menopause and give you continued or renewed youth for many years. And that is our goal.

Increased Sex Desire

The presence of female hormones will indirectly increase a woman's sexual desire. They do it through their action on the master pituitary gland at the base of the brain. They may even release you from apparent frigidity. But they will not cause excess sexual desire (nymphomania).

The increased sexual desire comes primarily from the fact that you remain more truly female as long as you do not see yourself "decaying" into the change of life neutral sex state. This makes you more ready and willing to play the female role, more ready and willing to take an active part in all sexual play.

You and Your Doctor Regarding Hormones

Let me tell you what to expect from your doctor when you become a candidate for the magical hormones. You should be given a complete physical examination. This is essential on general principles as well as to rule out any premalignant conditions. This examination should always include a pelvic and careful rectal study. Many precancerous conditions can be discovered in the early stages in this way, and easily corrected in the office.*

Your doctor will take a smear test from the mouth of the womb, not only for cancer, but also to determine the degree of femininity of your body. A special cell count shows this important warning signal of changing sex life and aging. If you are already in your menopause, the smear can be taken at any time, but if you are still menstruating, it should be taken between the twelfth and the fourteenth day of your cycle. Given the right clue, your physician can then start you on the magic hormones without delay, to either reverse or prevent the change of life aging.

How Many "Magic" Hormone Pills?

Once your doctor decides to put you on hormone treatment, once the deficiency is recognized, you need only swallow one tablet each day. On certain days of the month you may be told to swallow two tablets, or perhaps none at all.

You may see a little bleeding between periods. This is very common when you are taking the estrogens. It is also frequently seen by those women who are taking contraceptive pills. If you see it, your doctor will probably tell you to take a little more hormone at that time to keep your estrogen level where it belongs. He may want to advise two tablets each day for the rest of that cycle. Or he may want you to gradually increase your dose during each cycle. Follow his advice and do not panic if you see this little bleeding between periods while on the magic hormones.

How Women Can Choose Their Own Menstrual Cycle

Wonder of wonders, you can now choose your own menstrual cycle in many cases. Would you like to menstruate every seventy days? You can move this normal bleeding time backward or forward at will by varying the dosage schedule. Naturally, you will do exactly as your doctor advises. You understand that when your

---

* See my book, *Painless Office Rectal Treatment,* available from The UNITROL Teaching Institute. 147-41 Sanford Ave., Flushing, N.Y. 11355.

ovaries have stopped producing a balanced level of estrogens, you can juggle the pill hormone level and timing to suit your own convenience. This sex hormone treatment will not prolong the functioning of your ovaries, for this appears to be a pattern set down in your genes, and passed on from mother to daughter. In other words, the time when you enter the change of life is a set pattern determined before you were born. But once you have run out of natural hormone production, you can then be guided into a cyclical pattern of your own choice by adjusting the dosage and timing of the synthetic hormones.

Hormones and Pregnancy

Once you have entered the natural menopause, and your ovaries have stopped producing a correct hormone balance, you can take the synthetic hormones forever without any danger of becoming pregnant. You may continue to have regular menstrual periods— regular in the sense that they will occur at predetermined times regulated by the synthetic hormone dosage—without any danger of pregnancy.

It is probably best to give the hormones in regular cycles, perhaps for four weeks, and then withdraw them for seven to ten days to allow the lining of the uterus to shed (menstruation). This prevents excessive bleeding that might occur if the hormones were used continuously, without menstruation (due to excessive build-up of the lining of the womb).

With experience, we may find that many women will do quite well if they menstruate only four to six times a year. But this should be your physician's decision, and not yours.

The Hormones and Fibroids

Fibroid tumors of the womb are quite common. They may cause irregular or excessive bleeding, and sometimes they require surgical removal. But they tend to shrink after the menopause. When hormones are advised, some women seem to fear that their fibroid bleeding might be activated again. This is not the fact, and it is rarely a problem.

Both Birth and Age Control Possible Through Hormones

If you have been taking birth control pills, and have gone beyond the usual menopause time while still having your periods, it may well be that you have experienced both birth and age control at the same time! If you know when your mother began her change of life, and if you are now several years beyond that time, but still menstruating—and if you have been on birth control pills—this may be what is happening to you. Fine! Keep it up, and let yourself go sexually, since you are now on the path to "eternal" or constant youth without fear of undesired pregnancy.

This is due to the close chemical relationship between some birth control pills and the synthetic female hormones used for change of life treatment. In the usual change of life treatment, estrogen and progestin are given in sequence during the non-bleeding and the bleeding phases of the cycle. Most birth control pills, by contrast, contain both estrogen and progestin *in combination*. But it seems that if the birth control pills contain both estrogen and a *special estrogenic progestin*, you will be a candidate for both birth and automatic age control after the menopause. (Remember that not all of the birth control pills now on the market contain the *estrogenic* progestins. Some of the progestins may even be masculinizing in their action, and although they will prevent conception, they will not automatically give you age control after the menopause!)

The Neutral Sex—the "Third Sex"—
How to Prevent It Happening to You

With advancing age both sexes become more like each other, the female becoming less female and the male becoming less masculine. The result is the "neutral sex," neither feminine nor masculine. This third sex is seen most often around sixty years of age. The magic hormones may virtually eliminate the neutral third sex. We should think of both the female and the male change of life as deficiency disorders, and treat them with the magic hormones—the sex steroids. *New vigor and vitality, new youth can now be offered to both sexes.* This is not rejuvenation, but it is true revitalization. Combined with proper hormone and mineral-vitamin therapy, youth can be prolonged and life can be extended for many years.

The Male Menopause Reversed

After fifty, and often before, men enter a time of decreased sexual capacity. Often this is accompanied by fatigue, depression, and loss of interest in business as well as in life in general. There is a sense of impending death, a feeling that life has passed him by. That was the case of a fifty year old, prematurely aging patient, who found that he could no longer attain a satisfactory erection and had lost all pleasure in living.

I put him on the longevity diet, since his eating habits were not good, to say the least. The male sex hormones were then started, by injection, to determine the appropriate dosage for continuing use. He required one injection every two weeks, and the results were almost miraculous. His old vigor and interest in life were restored, and he said, "I am as good as I was twenty years ago!". At the time of this writing, years later, he still is.

"Age Reversal" Is Possible

The aging clock can even be turned back after you have begun to show the changes of aging. As you already know from our consultations on the First Key to Longevity, the cholesterol deposits in your arteries that age you may be removed by the proper diet to a great extent. It is now evident that the bone changes (loss of calcium) that occur after the menopause, can be corrected by the proper hormone treatment. And the dried out skin and vaginal tissues can be restored to normal. If you do not let the flabby breasts go too long without hormone treatment, you may be able to restore a firm tone to this important female tissue.

The prostate can be brought back to a more normal size, allowing the bladder to empty itself better. This may retard bladder and kidney infection and other damage, and, in some cases, even help in restoring a more normal level of blood pressure. And, let me repeat—a better hormone level will help your blood cholesterol level and your arteries to return to the condition of youth.

All of this is *age reversal, youth prolongation, and life extension.* All of this is yours if you turn the various Keys to Longevity as described and programmed in this book.

The Lazy Thyroid

There is still another magic hormone I want to tell you about. The thyroid gland lies at the base of the neck, and it secretes a magic hormone. If you have difficulty losing weight, even when you are on a very low caloric diet (seven hundred, perhaps), your problem may be an underactive thyroid gland. Your thyroid—and your general metabolism—may need the boost of the magical thyroid hormone.

This butterfly-shaped thyroid gland, weighing only about one ounce, controls your general body metabolism. It can be underactive or overactive. If it is underactive we call the condition hypothyroidism. Between 5 and 7 per cent of the general population have an underactive thyroid gland. These people do not think they are ill, but they do have a "tired, run-down feeling." They are overweight. Their hair thickens, their nails split, and they may be weak, nervous, and feel cold even in a warm room.

Case History of A Lazy Thyroid Normalized

This young lady—only 23—seemed always depressed. She was very constipated. Her weight was 40 pounds above the proper level for her age and skeletal structure. "I am always tired," she complained. Her skin was pale, coarse and cool. She showed all the other evidences of a lazy thyroid. A simple blood test (the protein-bound iodine test) showed that she did indeed have a lazy thyroid.

Treatment with the tiny thyroid analog pills (synthetic active thyroid hormone) completely reversed the picture, and released the lovely, alert youngster from her underactive metabolic cocoon. Premature aging had been brought to a halt, youthful vigor and vitality had been restored, and her life expectancy had been increased.

Have You "Lost Interest" in Life?

If you have lost interest in life, see what the protein-bound iodine test has to say about you. If you are no longer intrigued by sexual intercourse, and may even be trying to avoid it, you may be suffering from a lazy thyroid.

If you are always tired, nervous or run-down, the magic thyroid hormone may be "just what the doctor ordered."

If you are too fat, and do not respond to the usual diet control, you may not be the "diet cheat" your doctor thinks you are. You may have a metabolic problem, and you may need the thyroid hormone.

Tests for the Lazy Thyroid

There are several valuable tests for thyroid activity. The basal metabolism test is the best known, but I do not consider it to be as accurate as other tests. This is the method during which the patient breathes pure oxygen for a specified period of time. Various calculations are then made to determine how much oxygen is being used for each pound of body weight. If you have a sluggish thyroid, you will also have a low rate of oxygen consumption.

The P.B.I. (protein-bound iodine) test is simpler and more accurate. All that is needed is a small blood sample from an arm vein. The laboratory does the rest, and shows us a very accurate report on thyroid activity.

Another very simple test requires that you kneel on a chair while the doctor taps the back of one ankle just above the heel. The ankle jerk response is recorded on a strip of paper like an electrocardiograph device. This pattern seems to accurately measure thyroid function.

Still another test is a radioactive-iodine-uptake determination. The patient is given a radioactive iodine to swallow, and after a measured period of time (usually six to 24 hours), a scanner device measures the amount of radioactivity given off by the thyroid gland. This shows how your thyroid removes iodine from the blood stream and turns the iodine into the thyroid hormone. If your thyroid is underactive, you will retain the radioactive iodine in your thyroid gland for a longer than normal period of time.

But this test requires that you take the radioactive material into your body, and this is not altogether without objection. And false readings are possible.

There is still another test that does not require swallowing the radioactive material. In this test a small blood specimen is taken from an arm vein, and this specimen is then tested by contact with a radioactive material in a laboratory (the Trisorb test).

A minute or two in your doctor's office—a simple blood sample from an arm vein—and your thyroid activity can easily be determined by either the P.B.I. or the Trisorb test.

Treatment for Lazy Thyroid Is Simple

The treatment for a lazy thyroid is very simple. All you need do is swallow one or more tiny thyroid analog pills—once again, a magic hormone—each day. This will correct the deficiency disease of a lazy thyroid. This will restore your youth, vigor and vitality. This will help you melt away unwanted fat. This will return you to your normal, slender, vigorous and vivacious self.

And NOW, in summary . . .

Once again we come to the end of an important consultation. You have learned all about the Third Key to Longevity—the Magical Hormones. One of the best tips I can give you for renewed enjoyment of life—for renewed vigor and vitality—is to take advantage of this major advance in modern medicine. Once you replenish your supply of these vital hormones, you will see life differently. You will become a younger, happier and healthier person. You will be ready once again to take your seat at the banquet table of Life, to enjoy its infinite variety with every sense alert, with taste and sight and hearing and touch—all senses at the ready—to experience and feel and enjoy the pleasures and satisfactions of living.

1. Now you know that aging is largely a *deficiency* disease.
2. You have learned about the magic hormones, and you will be ready to use them to correct your deficiency, to prevent or to correct aging, and you can live a longer and healthier life.
3. You know that the magic hormones can keep a woman young in all her tissues, far beyond the menopause.
4. You know that there are male sex hormones to do the same for men.
5. You have learned that there are hormones that will control both pregnancy and aging at the same time!

6. You have learned what a hormone is, what the endocrine glands are, and how they do their vital work in your body.

7. The facts about these life regulators will help set you free from the menopausal deficiency disease changes.

8. You are now ready to become part of the modern sexual revolution.

9. You are now ready to start on the road to permanent youth.

10. You are now ready to take out the modern form of "heart insurance."

11. The facts about hormone cancer prevention and treatment will help you eliminate fear and overcome the cancer obstacle to longer life.

12. The third sex—the neutral sex—can now become a thing of the past.

13. In this consultation I have also introduced you to the lazy thyroid.

14. If you are overweight despite a limited diet, you now know the simple magic hormone treatment.

And so I leave you with the Third Key to Longevity—the Hormone Key, and welcome you to the land of eternal youth.

THE FOURTH KEY
TO LONGEVITY

CHAPTER 15

HOW "THINKING YOUNG" WILL GIVE YOU A LONGER AND HEALTHIER LIFE

You Are What You Think

To a very large extent you and I are what we think and what we eat. The First Key to Longevity has taught you what to eat if you wish to become younger and to live a long and productive life. The Fourth Key to Longevity will show you how to think young, for you must think the thoughts of youth if you are to remain young and healthy for your longer life.

When you think young, you will act young. As a man thinketh in his heart so is he. Think young and you will be young. Think old—think that you *are* old—and you will begin to walk slowly, your back will bow and bend, and your attitudes will be those of the aging.

Obviously, then, this is the Fourth Key to youth and longer life, and you must begin now to *think* and *act* young.

Associate with Youth as Much as Possible

The best way to keep the patterns of youth is to associate with the young. This will show you the new and ever-changing patterns of young thinking and behavior. Flexibility of thought and action is one of the attributes of youth. You must be ready to change at all times. You must change with the times. You can do this best if you spend as much time as possible with younger people.

Your Prior Patterns of Youth Versus Present Patterns of Aging

PPY is my code for the prior patterns of youth. PPA is my designation for the present patterns of aging. With the passage of time in your life there is a constant battle between the prior patterns of youth and the present patterns of aging, and youth loses to the aging processes in practically all cases! Few of us have the capacity for change, the flexibility of thought and behavior, to put up a winning battle.

But if you will follow the rules of the first Three Keys to Longevity, you will in fact remain internally younger despite the passage of time. Your physiological age will be younger than your chronological age. Now I am suggesting that you remain younger mentally as well—younger in your thinking patterns. And in this consultation I propose to tell you how to do this.

UNITROL: The Healing Magic of the Mind

If you have not yet read my book on UNITROL, I strongly urge you to do so as soon as you can. It will teach you all you need to know to contact and control the amazing powers of your subconscious mind. The release of the repressed energy of your subconscious mind will increase your general energy bank, give you infinitely greater control of your entire body than you have ever had, and will help you to reverse the aging processes. It will help you to achieve a happier and more satisfying life, and to overcome many of your PPA fears.

UNITROL does this primarily by showing you the inner workings of your subconscious mind, and by giving you conscious control over that powerful, but submerged fraction of your mind. I cannot give you the full techniques of UNITROL in a single consultation, and there is even more than appears in the book. Those of you who want to learn more about this amazing method for Unitary Control of your mind-body may write to me directly at the UNITROL Teaching Institute, 147-41 Sanford Ave., Flushing,

N.Y. 11355. You will receive a personal reply. When you write, please tell me of your progress with the Four Keys to Longevity.

How to Contact our Subconscious Constantly

I have hinted at contacting the subconscious when I told you to repeat—over and over again—while walking, the words—*younger and younger, younger and younger, younger and younger.*

Your subconscious mind accepts everything literally, and when you tell it, *"younger and younger,"* it will put into immediate action whatever body forces are necessary to achieve this end. You will find yourself walking with increasing bounce and vitality, increasing energy and zest, as your subconscious mind puts this command into action.

You need not tell your subconscious mind how to do it. It knows how, better than you do—even if you are a physician. After all, it has been keeping you breathing, your heart beating, your internal organs functioning reasonably well without any help from you (and often in spite of you) for many years!

The best contact is made when you are fully relaxed, and UNITROL teaches you how to achieve relaxation in depth. But you can do quite well by giving your subconscious mind the *younger and younger* command just before you fall off to sleep, and again as soon as you awaken in the morning. These are the best times to find your subconscious mind unguarded and relaxed and receptive, ready to receive and to act upon your positive, healing and youth-restoring suggestions.

PPY and Your Subconscious

Use this method to speak to your subconscious mind, and to implant positive, youth-restoring ideas during the times that you practice your Prior Patterns of Youth.

Let's look at some of these PPY's right now.

Dancing—a PPY

Dancing is one of the prior patterns of your youth. Dance as often as you can, whenever and wherever you can. Dance just for the sheer joy of it. Dance for fun. Dance for rhythmic body motions. Dance for exercise. Dance most of all just because you like to do it. If you never learned to dance, just move around in time to any type of music. You can even dance to the television commercials!

Dancing will release your muscles and joints from the locking effect of aging. Dancing will stir up your blood and increase the activity of your lungs and heart. Dancing will strengthen your heart. Dancing will help you achieve the lower blood cholesterol level of youth. Most of all—dancing, like smiling—*will make you happy.*

I have already taught you the method of dancing in bed, and have showed you how this will help you lose weight and slim your measurements. A slim, trim body is one of the best attributes of healthy youth.

Rope Skipping and Bicycle Riding

Refer back to the Second Key to Longevity (page 185), and you will find my instructions for real and imaginary rope skipping and both real and imaginary bicycle riding. These are PPY's of the best kind, since they are suitable for and accepted by all ages. Prize fighters skip rope, as do other athletes, to remain in good form. You may do the same, to remain young.

And as you ride your bike or skip your rope, or dance about the room, repeat to yourself, in rhythm with your motion—*younger and younger, younger and younger, younger and younger....* to bring your subconscious powers into action to mobilize the youth-producing hormones.

Hobbies—a Good PPY

An excellent PPY is a hobby. It does not matter what your hobby is, as long as *you* enjoy it. Collect sea shells, stamps, coins—whatever pleases you—to maintain an active interest in life. Your hobby may be both pleasant and profitable in some cases. It is largely up to you.

A very good hobby is to help others. You can do this as an individual or through an organization, church group, or civic group.

This is the best way to realize your human potential, to remain interested in life, to give of yourself. If you can afford it, give money. But best of all, give your services, your advice and guidance, and wisdom.

When you help others you will truly be helping yourself to become a more useful and better person. After all, this is one of the attributes of youth—interest in others, interest in life, and taking an active part in all of life's activities. This is a very wonderful PPY, fulfilling all our requirements for better living and a return to youth, even while benefiting from the wisdom of your experience and chronological age.

Painting and Sculpting

These are excellent creative activities. It is never too late to take up a creative art, and there are many places you can go to receive instruction—even without charge. Or you can become a "primitive" painter, as Grandma Moses did. Perhaps you have a talent you never recognized before, a talent that will give you satisfaction and possibly earn money for you.

Finger painting is a true PPY—really young. Try it for fun. It will make you feel young. Think young, act young, and you will be young. There are many PPY's that will occur to you, and—in moderation—try them all. The more you replace your PPA's with PPY's, the younger you will become.

Swinging in a Swing

Every public playground has swings both for youngsters and for older youngsters. You can be one of the older youngsters, if you like, and go swinging. This is a healthful PPY. Smile while you do it, and be happy. All your PPY's must be fun if they are to do you real good.

And always combine your PPY's with subconscious mind contact, giving the command, *younger and younger, younger and younger, younger and younger....* You will be surprised at how good you will feel after each of these PPY sessions, how much younger, how much more alert and vital.

Birthdays and Youth

Remain 29 all through your life. Whenever you celebrate your birthday let there be precisely 29 candles on your cake. Blow them out and make your wish. There is no need to grow older physiologically and mentally, even though time passes chronologically. Celebrate your 29th birthday when you are 100 and beyond.

This is the *PPY of 29*, and I want you to keep it forever. A good birthday wish is a command to your subconscious, given when you blow out the 29 candles: *Every day, in every way, I am becoming younger and younger, healthier and healthier, happier and happier.* Let your subconscious mind, and the Four Keys to Longevity, make it come true.

Think Happy Thoughts Always

It is important to keep positive, happy, *healing* thoughts in your mind. Remember that your subconscious mind acts without question on any suggestions you may give it, *good or bad*. Feed only happy thoughts, positive, *health-producing* suggestions to your very powerful subconscious mind. It is very important to be optimistic at all times, to have peace of mind, and to think happy thoughts. This is often more easily said than done, and that is why you should learn the simple methods of UNITROL to show you exactly how to achieve this very objective.

But until you do begin your practice of UNITROL, simply combine the *younger and younger* suggestion with every one of your PPY's.

Live NOW—There Is Only TODAY to DO IT

This is one of the best commandments I can give you. There is only today. Yesterday is gone, with all its mistakes and all its guilt— and good riddance. Tomorrow may never come. Besides, every tomorrow simply becomes another today. You must live today— RIGHT NOW—or you will not be living at all. Learn to see everything around you. Learn to hear all possible sounds. Learn to smell and feel and experience everything you possibly can.

A famous physician once commanded us to live each day in day-tight compartments. A still more famous man told us: "Sufficient unto the day are the cares thereof." Forget yesterday and tomorrow.

Live today—all of it! Don't die regretting that you never kissed "her" enough. Don't die regretting the things you never did. Do them now.

Travel—a PPY

The young like to get around. If you can travel to other countries you should do so without delay. If you can't afford the time or the money, you would be surprised to know how much there is to see and enjoy—with very little more than you already spend—right in your own home town. Look around and surprise yourself!

Stay Alert

Keep in contact with the world around you. There are amazing things going on all the time, and you can become part of them by knowing about them and talking about them. Don't spend your time talking about your aches and pains. Your subconscious mind will get every nuance of your thoughts and speech and will exaggerate your aches and pains for you. That is why it is so important to think happy thoughts and positive, health-giving suggestions all the time.

Read good, reliable newspapers and magazines. Read the latest books, the new authors. Take courses in adult education classes at the YMCA or YWCA, and in many other groups now readily available in practically every community.

Do you have a public library? The best minds of every generation are represented there, and they are all ready to welcome and instruct you. Make friends with books. They will help to keep you young.

Cut off General Anxiety Patterns

I recommend, on the other hand, that you cut off all communication with the general anxiety patterns, the fear and hate-mongers, the radio commentators who emphasize the evils of the world, the television programs and alarm-type newspapers that cater to sensation-seekers. They will upset your nervous system, and may even give you ulcers. This surely does not add up to a happy *long life*. As you think, so will you be—and I do not want you thinking destructive, evil, narrow, bigoted, or any other type of self-destructive thoughts. Love will extend and warm and make your life happy. Hate will shorten and freeze and destroy your life and your happiness. *Love one another* is a very great commandment.

UNTIL WE MEET AGAIN

And now, before you leave my consultation room, I want to take a few more moments to give you some additional tips on better health and longer life. These are the answers to questions that have been asked so often by those of my patients who are truly desirous of long life. I want to share them with you.

Sunshine—a Mixed Blessing

I remember visiting Florida to arrange a medical convention for the International Academy of Proctology. As I strolled along the beach, after my conferences in the hotel, I saw the sunworshippers stretched out on their "lounges" or on the sand, sunning first one side and then the other. Some were burnt red, some were deep brown, and others almost black. All were foolish. They had forgotten the rule of moderation.

They were sacrificing their future skin health for a present status symbol. In our society it is considered a sign of affluence to have a well tanned skin. But when you dry out your skin by excess exposure to sunlight, you are guaranteeing a rapidly aging skin in your later years. Excess sunshine makes your skin more susceptible to skin cancer. Moderation is your keynote, even when you take the life-giving sunshine on your skin.

Sunshine and Vision

Another serious mistake of the sun-worshipper is the fact that he invariably wears dark glasses to "protect" his eyes. Sunshine is essential for normal vision. Fish born and living in dark caves are blind. Without light there is no vision. Sunning the eyes—in moderation—is good for them, and strengthens vision. I do not mean that you should stare at the sun, for this will damage your sight. But you should not wear sunglasses. And you can even look toward the sun with your eyes closed, allowing the sun's rays to pass through your lids to work their healing magic on the optic nerves and on the retina.

Or you can look downward, with your eyes closed, as if you were straining to see your chin, and then hold your upper lids open with your index fingers, to let the sun safely warm and heal the eyeballs without injuring the delicate optic nerves. Do this for a few seconds each day, if you wish. It is especially beneficial if you are retraining your failing vision. For other eye-strengthening exercises you may wish to see my book, *Ridding Yourself of Psychosomatic Health Wreckers.*

Empty Bowel, Empty Bladder, Empty Brain (EB-EB-EB)

I call this the Essential Triad—essential for good health and long life. Regularity of the bowels is helped by proper diet combined with the type of exercise you have already learned about. The rolling of your abdominal muscles (see page 186), especially in the morning at the time of your regular bowel movement, will be very helpful in fully emptying your bowels.

It is important to realize that an empty bowel gives a sense of good health. Your large bowel has only one function—the absorption of water. If you do not drink enough water, your bowel wall will absorb the water from the stool itself. This leaves the stool hard and dry, and difficult to pass without injury to the outlet (fissure, ulcer, bleeding, and so on). This gives you still another good reason to drink at least six to eight glasses of water each day.

When you drink your daily water quota you will automatically keep your kidneys functioning to their best advantage. This will help you achieve the empty bladder that is so important to good health. Actually, the empty bladder merely symbolizes good kidney function, and this will become automatic when you eat the right foods and drink the right amount of water. The Longevity Diet will take care of both requirements.

But for the men, if your prostate gland is enlarged, you will need to follow your doctor's advice so that your bladder outlet will not be obstructed. Turn back to the section on the magic hormones (page 203), and you will find more information on control of an enlarging prostate.

Many years ago I wrote a paper with the tongue-twisting title, "The Hemorrhoidal-Prostatic-Impotence Syndrome." In this scientific paper I told of my observations relating hemorrhoids (varicose veins in the rectum) to an enlarged prostate and loss of virility. This was due to the pooling of blood in the prostate gland (since the varicose hemorrhoidal veins empty into the same group of veins that surround the prostate), causing a boggy and enlarged gland. And this, in turn, seemed to reduce sexual potency.

My experience showed that when the hemorrhoids were corrected by injections or removal, the prostate gland circulation improved and the gland returned to normal size. Potency was improved, in some cases to a surprising degree. Naturally, bladder emptying was also easier, since a boggy prostate usually partially obstructs the bladder outlet. This was corrected when the prostate became younger and firmer.

And Now—the Empty Brain

This is a big subject. Anxiety, the stress of everyday living, the frustrations of little things, the fear of the future and the guilt of the past, all contrive to distort and destroy our lives. If only we could empty the brain of the fears and frustrations, the guilt, the stress and anxiety! Fortunately we can! The method is called UNITROL, and you can see now why it is so important for you to read this book. It is essential for fulfillment of the final Key to Longevity— the control of the mind.

The search for self-knowledge and peace of mind is eternal, and UNITROL will put you on the path. When you have learned control of your body-mind *unit* (UNIT-TROL—the origin of the word), you will be able to rid yourself of the stress factors that shorten life, the guilt factors that prevent true enjoyment of life, and the psychosomatic health wreckers that cry out with the organ language of distressed tissues and body systems. You will have emptied your brain of its emotional garbage, and released its energies for creative living, better health and longer life with renewed youth.

Zen Wisdom

I have already introduced you to the poem:

> *Inch time*
> *Foot gem*

This is profound wisdom, teaching us that a single moment of time is worth more than a priceless gem. And yet how many of us sell our souls for money! How many of us grow old before our time in the pursuit of fortune and fame, worn out and used by ambition! You must change your way of thinking if you are to free yourself from enslavement to ambition, to the struggle for more and more money. If you seek early death and a tombstone that reads:

He Lived—He Made Money—He Died

keep on just as you are. But if you really understand the wisdom of *Inch time, Foot gem,* then you will not sell a single moment of your life for any price.

Most of my patients are not wealthy, but some are millionaires. I have yet to find a single millionaire who would trade his wealth for better health and longer life! Astonished? You shouldn't be, for they became millionaires by trading their lives for money. They had already determined their sense of values, and would not change even on their death beds. You must decide for yourself whether or not to live by the wisdom of *Inch time, Foot gem.*

The Lessons of the Hunzas for Healthful Long Life

Many of my patients are familiar with the fact that the Hunzas live very long active lives, and they ask me if I know the Hunza secret. I do.

The fabulous Hunzakuts, in their Himalayan mountain valley, have important lessons to teach those of us who wish to live 100 or more years. These people often live well beyond 100, have little or no heart disease, and no cancer. It is said that the men father children after they have passed the ninety-year mark. They can run great distances, dance for hours, and have enormous vitality.

How did they get that way? First, of course, is the genetic factor —the type of tissue they were born with—and there is nothing you or I can do about that. We are what we are, and we must do the best we can with the body tissues God gave us.

But there are some factors that can be controlled, and the people of Hunza land give us some important clues. *First,* they work hard all their lives—outdoors, and usually in the fields. *Second,* they play hard—dance with pleasure and grace. *Third,* they eat very little, and at certain seasons of the year, when the food supply is scarce, they actually fast for a period. *Fourth,* they eat little meat, since meat is always scarce. *Fifth,* their crops are grown without chemical fertilizers or insecticides. *Sixth,* they eat only natural foods with all their natural vitamins and minerals—not the processed, chemically treated foods of our civilization. *Seventh,* they drink the mineral-rich waters of their glacier-fed streams. *Eighth,* they have no possessions to steal, and no desire for more than they need. There is practically no crime and no juvenile delinquency in their land.

In simple terms and in summary—they live without the stress, frustration and guilt of our "enlightened" civilization, and they live close to the soil.

No coronary killers, none of the C factors of coronary disease; that, in brief, is the secret of Hunza land. And that, my friend, is the secret of our Longevity Program, as you have learned it throughout our consultations.

And NOW, in final summary . . .

In our final consultation I have taught you the Fourth Key to Longevity. But this is a lifelong study, and I have directed you to other books so that you may really apply the methods and the wisdom of self-knowledge to help you turn the Key of Thought to unlock the inner door to better health and longer life. You have learned that . . .

1. You are what you think and what you eat.
2. You have learned how to think young.
3. When you think young you will act young and you will become younger.
4. You have learned why you must associate with youth.
5. I have taught you the PPY's and how to use them to combat the PPA's.
6. I have introduced you to the importance of UNITROL.

7. I have taught you a simple method to contact your sub-conscious, and to enlist it in your search for youth and longer life.
8. I have instructed you in the importance of continuing flexibility and creativity, and have showed you how to use this instruction to stay young in mind and body.
9. I have given you the all-important NOW therapy.
10. I have offered more tips to better, healthier and longer living—tips that you can use right NOW.
11. I have introduced you to the vital EB,EB,EB concept—the Essential Triad.
12. I have given you the wisdom of Zen, and the secret of the Hunzas.

INDEX